362.1 RES
Resnik, David B.
Dying declarations

c.1

DATE DUE

JUL 01 2009			
FEB 05 2014			
JUL 07 2018			

El Segundo Public Library

David B. Resnik, JD, PhD

Dying Declarations
Notes from a Hospice Volunteer

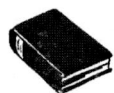

**Pre-publication
REVIEWS,
COMMENTARIES,
EVALUATIONS . . .**

"**D**r. Resnik has given us a wonderful collection of stories that illustrate the richness of the experience of living with dying. He takes his readers on a journey into the lives of hospice patients and their families as he shares his experiences as their hospice volunteer. The reader will come away with a sense of the gifts that can come from sharing this special time of life with dying people and their loved ones. I recommend this book to anyone who may be considering being a hospice volunteer."

Susan Redding, MSN, FNP-C
*Clinical Nurse Specialist
for Advance Care Planning
and End of Life Care,
Pitt County Memorial Hospital,
End of Life Care Program*

"**I**n *Dying Declarations,* David Resnik writes of his own experience and growth as a hospice volunteer. His touching and personal stories of patients illustrate the unique qualities of the lives he touched, and they capture the broad range of needs of hospice clients and their families. He is instructive through the lens of his own experience—each person teaching him some sort of lesson about people or life itself.

This book is a pleasant read and would be helpful to someone considering becoming a hospice volunteer. Prospective volunteers often wonder what the role is really like and how one learns to feel at ease working with people at the end of life. David Resnik addresses these questions up front. He writes about bringing one's skills as a *person* to the hospice experience, and his stories reassure us that those qualities, when sincerely given, are a gift indeed."

Margaret Franckhauser, ARNP
*Executive Director,
Community Health & Hospice, Inc.,
Laconia, New Hampshire*

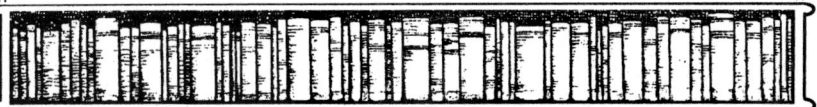

More pre-publication
REVIEWS, COMMENTARIES, EVALUATIONS . . .

"Providing hospice care is a philosophy of support for people who are dying and their loved ones. Death is a natural part of life. Hospice care is about dignity at this most profound stage of life; it is about the human condition and how the very simple things such as sharing time together, listening, talking, doing chores, or going shopping can make a difference in the lives of those who are dying and their primary caregivers.

Dr. Resnik has written a compassionate book that celebrates people's lives as well as illustrating the basic but wonderful support that hospice volunteers provide. The writing is easy for the reader even though the messages at times are quite profound. Readers will benefit immensely from this book because the window that is opened on other people's lives is also a mirror on our own.

Dr. Resnik has provided the reader a narrative on many of the hospice volunteer relationships he has had over the years. He feels he has benefitted much more from these relationships than those who received his help. We should feel similarly privileged as he gives us a glimpse of the way death and dying is approached. It is one man's pause for reflection on life, and it serves as a lesson for living for anyone that reads this book."

Malcolm Anderson, PhD
Visiting Research Fellow,
The Change Foundation;
Assistant Professor, Department
of Physical Medicine and Rehabilitation,
Faculty of Health Sciences,
Queen's University,
Kingston, Canada

"Through his creative use of storytelling, David Resnik is able to provide the reader with a glimpse into the reality of the lives of those who have touched his life in hospice palliative care. As difficult as this may be, his is able to account for their unique reality without judgment, and at the same time share his own experience and lessons learned from the incredible people who have touched his life. David touches on many sensitive issues in hospice palliative care as he carefully chooses his stories to illuminate the many dilemmas that people face at end of life. Many face very difficult choices that have a great impact on their quality of life and the lives of their family and friends. David demonstrates through his stories the value of living in the moment and being present for these individuals who appreciate being heard, needing to tell their stories in their own way without fear of being judged or told what to do.

This is a great handbook for anyone who is interested in or currently working with individuals at end of life. The techniques that Resnik describes are ones that can be used by others in a variety of different settings but especially those who work in hospice palliative care. Volunteers are the wind beneath the wings of hospice and this book is a wonderful example of the value that a volunteer brings to this area of practice and especially to individuals at end of life."

Filomena Nalewajek, MN, RN
Executive Director,
Canuck Place Children's Hospice,
Vancouver, British Columbia

More pre-publication
REVIEWS, COMMENTARIES, EVALUATIONS . . .

"Dr. Resnik shares his experience with loss, both personal and as a hospice volunteer, in fourteen stories. Eleven are encounters with perfect strangers and their families. One is about the death of his own grandmother, another the untimely loss of his wife's cousin, and finally the heartwrenching experience of putting the family dog Pepper to sleep after seemingly endless years of companionship. He witnessed great distresses such as denial, regret, guilt, sorrow, anger, loneliness, uncertainty, helplessness, anxiety, and injustice, but he also encountered unconditional love, selflessness, bravery, stoicism, forgiveness, acceptance, respect, appreciation, kindness, devotion, caring, and gratitude.

After reading these stories, we reflect and tell ourselves to slow down, smell the roses, taste the lemonade, and take care of ourselves and ours. Be there for each other. In the end, running errands, chopping wood, cleaning house, providing respite, making a sandwich, lending an attentive ear, playing music or a board game, reading the Bible, and recording one's legacy turn out to be those little onerous chores that can be so meaningful and enhance the quality of life for the dying and their families.

By helping and serving our fellow human in such seemingly minor or trivial ways, we relieve anxiety, provide peace of mind, reduce caregiver burnout, and allow the dying to feel valued and connected to the human condition. In return, we regain our own humanity. We gain much by appreciating our family and our health. We are grateful for what we have and are less troubled by what we don't. Our perspective of what matters most and our priorities on what is important in life are often reset. We become less judgmental. Perhaps we become better prepared for our own mortality and learn how to accept our own losses—past, present, and future.

I enjoyed the book. It read easily. I would recommend it to any health care professionals who care for patients near the end of life. Any professionals who enjoy knowing their patients as people with illnesses will find these stories meaningful and remind them of why they pursued a career in medicine. Finally, any people wishing to do hospice work or to be hospice volunteers, but are undecided, will find this book helpful in decision making."

George Ho Jr., MD
Professor of Medicine,
Brody School of Medicine,
East Carolina University,
Greenville, North Carolina

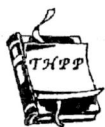

The Haworth Pastoral Press®
An Imprint of The Haworth Press, Inc.
New York • London • Oxford

NOTES FOR PROFESSIONAL LIBRARIANS AND LIBRARY USERS

This is an original book title published by The Haworth Pastoral Press®, an imprint of The Haworth Press, Inc. Unless otherwise noted in specific chapters with attribution, materials in this book have not been previously published elsewhere in any format or language.

CONSERVATION AND PRESERVATION NOTES

All books published by The Haworth Press, Inc. and its imprints are printed on certified pH neutral, acid-free book grade paper. This paper meets the minimum requirements of American National Standard for Information Sciences-Permanence of Paper for Printed Material, ANSI Z39.48-1984.

362.1 RES
Resnik, David B.
Dying declarations
c.1

Dying Declarations
Notes from a Hospice Volunteer

THE HAWORTH PASTORAL PRESS®
Religion and Mental Health
Harold G. Koenig, MD
Senior Editor

A Theology of God-Talk: The Language of the Heart by J. Timothy Allen

A Practical Guide to Hospital Ministry: Healing Ways by Junietta B. McCall

Pastoral Care for Post-Traumatic Stress Disorder: Healing the Shattered Soul by Daléne Fuller Rogers

Integrating Spirit and Psyche: Using Women's Narratives in Psychotherapy by Mary Pat Henehan

Chronic Pain: Biomedical and Spiritual Approaches by Harold G. Koenig

Spirituality in Pastoral Counseling and the Community Helping Professions by Charles Topper

Parish Nursing: A Handbook for the New Millennium edited by Sybil D. Smith

Mental Illness and Psychiatric Treatment: A Guide for Pastoral Counselors by Gregory B. Collins and Thomas Culbertson

The Power of Spirituality in Therapy: Integrating Spiritual and Religious Beliefs in Mental Health Practice by Peter A. Kahle and John M. Robbins

Bereavement Counseling: Pastoral Care for Complicated Grieving by Junietta Baker McCall

Biblical Stories for Psychotherapy and Counseling: A Sourcebook by Matthew B. Schwartz and Kalman J. Kaplan

A Christian Approach to Overcoming Disability: A Doctor's Story by Elaine Leong Eng

Faith, Medicine, and Science: A Festschrift in Honor of Dr. David B. Larson edited by Jeff Levin and Harold G. Koenig

Encyclopedia of Ageism by Erdman Palmore, Laurence Branch, and Diana Harris

Dealing with the Psychological and Spiritual Aspects of Menopause: Finding Hope in the Midlife by Dana E. King, Melissa H. Hunter, and Jerri R. Harris

Spirituality and Mental Health: Clinical Applications by Gary W. Hartz

Dying Declarations: Notes from a Hospice Volunteer by David B. Resnik

Maltreatment of Patients in Nursing Homes: There Is No Safe Place by Diana K. Harris and Michael L. Benson

Is There a God in Health Care? Toward a New Spirituality of Medicine by William F. Haynes and Geffrey B. Kelly

Guide to Ministering to Alzheimer's Patients and Their Families by Patricia A. Otwell

The Unwanted Gift of Grief: A Ministry Approach by Tim P. Van Duivendyk

Dying Declarations
Notes from a Hospice Volunteer

David B. Resnik, JD, PhD

The Haworth Pastoral Press®
An Imprint of The Haworth Press, Inc.
New York • London • Oxford

For more information on this book or to order, visit
http://www.haworthpress.com/store/product.asp?sku=5259

or call 1-800-HAWORTH (800-429-6784) in the United States and Canada
or (607) 722-5857 outside the United States and Canada

or contact orders@HaworthPress.com

Published by

The Haworth Pastoral Press®, an imprint of The Haworth Press, Inc., 10 Alice Street, Binghamton, NY 13904-1580.

© 2005 by The Haworth Press, Inc. All rights reserved. No part of this work may be reproduced or utilized in any form or by any means, electronic or mechanical, including photocopying, microfilm, and recording, or by any information storage and retrieval system, without permission in writing from the publisher. Printed in the United States of America.

PUBLISHER'S NOTE
Some identities and circumstances of individuals discussed in this book have been changed to protect confidentiality.

Cover design by Kerry E. Mack.

Library of Congress Cataloging-in-Publication Data

Resnik, David B.
   Dying declarations : notes from a hospice volunteer / David B. Resnik.
     p. cm.
   Includes bibliographical references and index.
   ISBN-13: 978-0-7890-2544-9 (hard : alk. paper)
   ISBN-13: 978-0-7890-2545-6 (pbk. : alk. paper)
   ISBN-10: 0-7890-2544-2 (hard : alk. paper)
   ISBN-10: 0-7890-2545-0 (pbk. : alk. paper)
   1. Hospice care—Anecdotes. 2. Terminal care—Anecdotes. 3. Palliative treatment—Anecdotes. 4. Dying—Anecdotes. 5. Volunteer workers in terminal care. I. Title.

R726.8.R467 2005
616'.029—dc22

                                                                   2004026631

The book is dedicated to the patients
I have known as a hospice volunteer,
their families, and health care professionals
everywhere that take care of patients
who are near the end of life.

ABOUT THE AUTHOR

David B. Resnik, JD, PhD, is Adjunct Professor of Philosophy and Religion at North Carolina State University. He previously served in the Department of Medical Humanities at the Brody School of Medicine at East Carolina University. He has published more than 100 articles on philosophy and ethics and is the author of *The Ethics of Science: An Introduction*; *Human Germ-line Gene Therapy: Scientific, Moral, and Political Issues*; and *Responsible Conduct in Research*. He is also the Associate Editor of the journal *Accountability in Research* and is on the Board of Directors for the North Carolina Association for Biomedical Research. His current research interests are in ethical issues in biomedical research, biotechnology and human genetics, and philosophical issues in science, technology, and medicine. Dr. Resnik has volunteered for hospices and nursing homes since 1995.

CONTENTS

Preface	ix
Chapter 1. Hospice Training	1
Chapter 2. We Need to Get Some Wood in Before Winter	7
Chapter 3. One M&M at a Time	13
Chapter 4. See the World While You Can	17
Chapter 5. I Have a Dream	21
Chapter 6. I Can Fix It	27
Chapter 7. Piggly Wiggly Has the Best Service	31
Chapter 8. Give Yourself Some Living Room	37
Chapter 9. Plant a Garden	41
Chapter 10. I Need to Go to Church	49
Chapter 11. I Knew You Were Okay When I Saw You Pull Up in a Ford Truck	53
Chapter 12. You Don't Know All the Bad Things I've Done	59
Chapter 13. He Was a Helluva Ballplayer	65
Chapter 14. Euthanasia	71
Bibliography	79
Index	81

Preface

This book is a collection of stories, observations, and reflections based on my relationships with people who are dying. The book is about what I have learned from these people, and what they can teach all of us about living. Most of the book draws on my experiences as a volunteer for hospices and nursing homes from 1995 through 2003. I have changed all the names of patients I have known and some of the facts about their stories in order to protect their privacy. I have not changed the names of dying relatives that I have known.

I chose the title *Dying Declarations* from an unusual part of the law on evidence in criminal and civil trials. For many years, the U.S. legal system has had various prohibitions on hearsay testimony, which can be defined as "an out-of-court statement used to prove the truth of the matter asserted." If an individual on the witness stand testifies that "John said that he was a careful driver," then this statement will not be admitted to prove that John was a careful driver, unless a particular hearsay exception allows the testimony to be admitted. The law on hearsay is a complex labyrinth of rules, exceptions, exclusions, and privileges, each of which can be bent or interpreted to meet some particular purpose.

Tucked away in the middle of this maze lies a rule with a human face. The rule on "dying declarations" allows the statement of a dying person to be admitted as testimony in a court of law if the dying person (1) is not now available to testify, (2) believed that his or her death was imminent when making the statement, and (3) made the statement about the cause of his or her death. The theory behind this hearsay exception, according to the *Federal Rules of Evidence* (2002), is that someone who believes that death is imminent is likely to give reliable testimony. Dying people have very few reasons to lie and many reasons to tell the truth.

People who are in the process of dying have a great deal to teach us, if we will only listen. They can teach us about making the most of each day and about being fully present in the moment. They can teach us about being patient with ourselves and with other people. They can teach us about what has been meaningful to them in their lives and what is meaningful in our lives. They can teach us about what they fear and regret and what we may fear or regret. They can teach us about the importance of friendship, love, service, dreams, memories, and hope.

I started serving as a volunteer in hospices and nursing homes after my grandmother, Muriel Resnik, died in February 1995. Muriel (or "Mumu") was a petite woman with wavy auburn hair, pensive brown eyes, a sharp wit, and a flair for the dramatic. She was a writer and an adventurer. She wrote books and plays, including the Broadway hit *Any Wednesday*. She traveled extensively and was an excellent cook. She loved Italian food, waterfronts, historic houses, Mel Brooks movies, and fresh vegetables.

We had a close relationship. I saw her when my family visited her, but I also went by myself to visit her in New York City, Stony Creek, Connecticut, and Beaufort, North Carolina. We wrote letters. She took me on trips, to movies, and to restaurants; she took me to FAO Schwarz. She gave me some of her favorite Beatles records. And most of all, she encouraged me to write. A "writer writes," she would say. It has been eight years since she died, and I still miss her.

Mumu was in very good health for many years and had a great deal of youthful vigor. She exercised, ate health foods, stopped smoking in the 1960s, and drank only in moderation. We had a birthday party for her when she was seventy-five years old—officially, she never told us her age—and we fully expected that she would live to be 100. Her mother had lived into her nineties, and she had an aunt that lived to be 101 years old.

Mumu had arthritis for many years. For a long time, she was able to keep the disease at bay by walking her two terriers every day, swimming, and eating well. Mumu's arthritis got much worse, and she became unable to walk her dogs. Her doctor prescribed a powerful anticancer drug, methatrexate, to treat her arthritis. The drug made her very ill, and she couldn't stand taking it. She would wait until her arthritis flared up to take the drug. Not long after she started taking methatrexate, she developed a crippling, neuromuscular degenerative disease. She might have developed this disease even if she had not taken methatrexate, but it is also possible that the drug triggered the disease. My wife, Susan, who is a pharmacist, was opposed to her taking this drug, but we were powerless to intervene in Mumu's situation.

Mumu's muscles got weaker and weaker. She developed shingles, and her arthritis got worse. Soon she couldn't walk and she had trouble eating, talking, and swallowing. She left her adopted home in Beaufort for the security and familiarity of her apartment in New York. She became depressed. She spent all of her time in her bedroom, with the curtains drawn. She did not want to believe that she was gravely ill, and she talked as if she would recover soon. She developed a life-threatening area of fluid in her brain that needed to be drained with a shunt. She did not want to have the shunt placed in her head, because this would mean acknowledging that she was seriously ill. Eventually, she relented.

We were living in Wyoming at the time, and it was difficult for us to visit any of our family, most of whom lived in North Carolina. During our visit to North Carolina in December 1994, we decided to fly to New York with our son, Peter, to visit Mumu. We saw her only twice during our visit; she was too tired and in too much pain to have many visitors. We found her all alone in a dark room—moaning, crying, and emaciated.

I stayed with Mumu for a while and we talked. Because she was very weak, I did most of the talking. We talked about our common memories and about the good times we had. We talked about our trip to Greece and Italy when I was ten years old. We talked about the summer that I helped out with her bed-and-breakfast in Beaufort. We talked about her disease and her suffering. We talked about Susan and Peter and the future. We did not talk about death or the fact that she was dying. It is obvious to me now that she was dying, and that she probably should have had hospice care, but no one, including her doctor, was facing up to this fact at the time. We were going through Elisabeth Kübler-Ross's (*On Death and Dying,* 1997) well-documented stage of grief known as denial.

Mumu's husband, Victor Jackson, made heroic efforts to care for her during her final months of life. He was her nurse, cook, maid, and chauffeur. He bathed her, fed her, and comforted her. He took her to the doctor and kept track of all of her medications. The day that she died, he carried her down the stairs and rushed her to the hospital, but it was to no avail. Because they had not prepared for her to die at home, he could not let her die in the apartment. She did not have a "do-not-resuscitate order."* The doctors were still trying to "do everything" for her. But everything wasn't enough.

I felt great sorrow when Mumu died. I wept; I reminisced; I wrote; and I rationalized. After these feelings passed, I began to feel anger, the next stage in dealing with death. I was angry that she died so soon. I thought she would be around for at least another decade. I also was angry at the way she died. Why did she have to die like this? If there are any "good deaths," hers was not one of them.

Uncontrolled anger is a terrible thing, but anger properly channeled toward a good cause can be a wonderful thing. The acronym for Mothers Against Drunk Driving, MADD, is a perfect example of properly channeled anger. My anger at Mumu's death motivated me to take an interest in hospice and in working with dying people. What Mumu really needed during her final months of life was a friend, but I was 2,000 miles away. I thought I could relieve my guilt and redeem her death by helping other people have better final days.

In my experience as a hospice volunteer, I have found that many other volunteers have been motivated to help dying patients as a result of powerful experiences with dying relatives or friends.

---

*A do-not-resuscitate (DNR) order is an order written by a physician not to use resuscitative measures, such as cardiopulmonary resuscitation (CPR), on a patient. DNR orders can be written in a hospital or nursing home setting. Most states also recognize out-of-hospital (or community) DNR orders, which apply to the home environment. Most hospice patients that I have worked with have had out-of-hospital DNR orders, although this is not a requirement for hospice care.

Some, like me, decided to work with dying people as the result of a bad experience. Others decided to undertake this service as a result of a good experience, usually with hospice.

Before concluding this preface, I would like to thank Georganne Perry, for reading drafts of the manuscript, and my wife, Susan Resnik, for encouragement and helpful discussions.

I should also confess that my interests in dying people are academic and professional as well as personal. I have taught courses in bioethics since I was a graduate student in philosophy at the University of North Carolina. I have studied the philosophical, moral, legal, and theological aspects of death and dying. In my current role as a professor of medical humanities at The Brody School of Medicine at East Carolina University, I teach medical students, medical residents, and hospital staff about ethical and legal issues in health care; I consult on ethics cases; and I serve on ethics committees.

This book is therefore a kind of experiment for me in the art of bridging the gap between moral theory and moral practice. I have never been happy with this inherent gap, and I have tried to bridge it in my relationships with people. My work in hospice has been a personal application of ethical principles to particular situations, and writing about this work has allowed me to bridge the gap between theory and practice. Thought and action come together in the written or spoken word.

Although this book records my experiences, observations, and thoughts, it is not really about me. I have written this book to honor the memory of the people who have taught me so much. It is their story that I feel compelled to tell. Each one of these people had a dying declaration, and I would like to help tell it.

Chapter 1

Hospice Training

I learned about hospice in 1991 while teaching bioethics at the University of Wyoming. Our readings on end-of-life decisions presented two diametrically opposed positions: one can relieve suffering in terminally ill patients through euthanasia/assisted suicide, or one can force patients to continue living and suffering. In our class discussion, one of my students, an older woman who had returned to school after twenty years with the police force, mentioned that hospice care is a third alternative to these polarized views. She explained to the group how hospice helps people die with dignity and comfort but does not endorse euthanasia or assisted suicide. This was the first time I had heard about hospice care, and I was eager to learn more.

The hospice movement emerged in the late 1960s in the United Kingdom as an alternative to high-tech interventions at the end of life. Hospice is more than a place, a treatment, or an organization: it is a philosophy of caring for dying patients and their loved ones. Hospice is for dying patients who are forgoing curative medical care in favor of comfort and dignity at the end of life. The hospice approach provides dying patients with pain control and palliation, nursing care, occupational or physical therapy, and emotional and spiritual support. Hospice also offers family members respite care, bereavement counseling, and emotional and spiritual support. Hospice opposes active euthanasia, suicide, or other measures designed to shorten life (Beresford, 1993).

The hospice approach is palliative, not curative. It encourages patients and families to accept death as a natural part of life and to make the most of the time that remains. Hospice emphasizes individualized care and patient autonomy; patients and their families are free to decide what constitutes a "a dignified death." For more information on this concept, I recommend *What Dying People Want* (Kuhl, 2002), *The Grace in Dying* (Singh, 1998), *The Good Death* (Webb, 1997), *Dying Well* (Byock, 1997), *How We Die* (Nuland, 1994), and *Final Gifts* (Kelley and Callahan, 1992).

Many hospice patients choose to die at home, surrounded by friends and family members. However, for some patients dying at home is not an option. For these patients, hospice care can be provided in a nursing home or hospital setting. Some hospice patients spend some or most of their time in freestanding hospice facilities.

Hospice care was not always as professionalized or organized as it is today. At one time, hospice care was provided by local networks of volunteers and health care providers with a commitment to caring for patients at the end of life. Before the 1990s, most health insurers, including Medicare, did not pay for hospice care. (The Medicare hospice benefit applies to patients who have been diagnosed with six months or less to live and who have chosen to refuse curative care and to seek palliative care only.) Hospice care was supported through private donations of time and money, as well as payments from patients. It was a more informal and volunteer operation.

Today, hospice care is organized, professionalized, and, for the most part, adequately financed. Health insurers and Medicare pay for hospice care. Most hospice care today takes place through a hospice agency, which is a health care organization licensed by the state and by accrediting agencies, such as the Joint Commission on the Accreditation of Healthcare Organizations. The hospice agency may be associated with a home health agency or hospital system.

Hospice takes a multidisciplinary approach to patient care. A typical hospice team includes doctors, nurses, nurses' aides, pharmacists, social workers, and occupational and physical therapists. Volunteers also play an important role in hospice care. For more information on hospice, browse the Web site of the National Hospice and Palliative Care Organization at <http://www.nhpco.org/templates/1/homepage.cfm>.

Although I became aware of hospice care after learning about it through my bioethics teaching, I did not decide to become a hospice volunteer until a couple of months after Mumu died. In May 1995, I signed up for hospice and attended a training session for volunteers. The training session took place on a Saturday. We listened to presentations from a physician, a couple of nurses, some clergy, and a social worker. They provided us with information on the hospice philosophy; pain and symptom control; chronic and terminal illnesses; active listening; signs and symptoms of patients who are dying; bereavement and the five stages of grief (denial, anger, depression, bargaining, acceptance); patient and volunteer safety (e.g., minimizing the risks of falls or injury and transmission of infectious diseases); confidentiality; religious beliefs about death and dying; spirituality and the dying process; and what hospice volunteers can and cannot do. I was deeply moved by the stories they had to tell and by their enthusiasm for their work. Since becoming a volunteer, I have attended other training sessions and participate in continuing education.

One of the ideas that most impressed me during my training was that of active listening. I was told that we have two ears and one mouth for a reason: we should listen twice as much as we talk. What many patients and family members need is simply someone who will listen and pay attention. Active listening requires the listener to ask questions that invite the speaker to talk more. One can ask questions in a friendly way without prying into someone's affairs. Most people want to talk, especially about themselves.

Active listening also requires one not to judge the patient but to hear what the patient has to say and to be a sounding board for the patient's own concerns. Sometimes it is not easy to listen without judging. Some patients may talk about bad things that have happened to them or that they have done to other people. Some patients may express their prejudices against specific racial or ethnic groups or religious creeds. Although it is tempting to admonish the patient for past or present misdeeds, one should try to avoid doing this. I have found it much more useful to simply repeat to the patient what he or she said in his or her own words. This allows the patient to judge his or her own words and deeds, without input from the volunteer.

Obviously, one of the most important things that a volunteer can do for a patient or the patient's family is to listen. Health care professionals, even those who work for hospice agencies, often do not have enough time to listen to patients. A typical hospice nurse may need to see five to seven patients in one day, and often does not have enough time to take care of the patient's physical needs *and* to listen. Good listening (and talking) requires ample free time—time when there is nothing better to do than have a conversation.

Ironically, family members and friends may also find it difficult to listen to their dying loved ones. Very often, family members are physically, emotionally, and spiritually exhausted from taking care of the patient for many months or years. They may have their own "issues" with the patient, such as unresolved anger or jealousy. For some, it is difficult to hear the same story or concern that one has heard for many years. Dementia, which is a common problem with many dying patients, can exacerbate this problem; the patient may be repeating a comment for the tenth time that day.

Even clergy, the people who are supposed to know how to listen, may not be the best listeners at times. Many clergy do a very good job of listening, but others like to talk, gossip, sermonize, or pray. Many patients are uncomfortable sharing their secrets, apprehensions, and regrets with a minister, priest, or rabbi, because they fear that they will be judged. Many patients do not want to admit to a man or woman of God that they are not sure whether they believe in God.

This is where hospice volunteers can provide a very unique and important service for dying patients and their families. Unlike health care providers, hospice volunteers have enough time to listen to the patient. Although it seems that everyone leads a very busy life today, hospice volunteers are not on a schedule where they must visit a specific number of patients each day. A volunteer will usually be assigned only one patient at a time. He or she may visit the patient once a week for a couple of hours, at most. If a volunteer can make time in his or her schedule to visit a hospice patient, then the volunteer will usually have enough time to listen.

Unlike family members or friends, hospice volunteers have no prior life experiences with the patient that could lead to unresolved anger, disappointment, jealousy, or emotional or spiritual exhaustion. They have not heard the same stories (or worries) a thousand times. Unlike clergy, hospice volunteers have no previous religious or spiritual history with the patient that could lead the patient to believe that he or she is being judged. A hospice volunteer is a fresh face with a new perspective.

Before I became a hospice volunteer, I had mistaken ideas about hospice. I thought that providing hospice care would be depressing, draining, and frustrating, since the patients are usually very sick, suffering, and dying. I would need to be a moral saint in order to bear such a demanding task. Many people I have talked to about being a hospice volunteer also think of this service as sheer martyrdom.

My preconceived ideas turned out to be completely wrong. I have found that serving as a hospice volunteer is uplifting, invigorating, and rewarding. Being a hospice volunteer has helped me to better appreciate the value of life and the importance of human relationships. It has helped me to learn to treasure each day and each person. Death strips away all of the superficial and mundane details of living and leaves behind life's bare essentials. By facing death on a regular basis, one can no longer maintain a tight grip on the masks, games, and trivialities that one uses to hide from the truth. The person who looks death in the eye becomes more honest, grateful, compassionate, and humble.

Sometimes I think I benefit much more from serving as a hospice volunteer than patients and families benefit from my help. I feel privileged and honored to be a part of their private, emotional, and sacred encounters with death and dying.

Chapter 2

We Need to Get Some Wood in Before Winter

After completing my hospice training, I was supposed to be ready for my first assignment. Yet none of my training prepared me for what it was really like to go into the house of a total stranger, a person who was dying. It's difficult enough to meet new people; meeting new people who are going through a difficult time is even more so. What should I say? What should I do? How could I help? What if someone starts to cry? When should I leave?

Before becoming a hospice volunteer, I had very little experience with talking to anyone about death and dying. Although our culture has made a great deal of progress in discussing the subject of death, it can still be an awkward subject. For many people, it is easier to talk about sex, politics, or religion.

Because I was not accustomed to talking to people about death and dying, I had to learn how to do this, which meant that I had to practice doing it. I have found that there is no simple formula for discussing death with people except to actively listen and to say and do what comes naturally. Because every one of us will die someday, we share a common bond in our fear of death. It is this commonality that enables people from very different religious, ethnic, and cultural backgrounds to talk about death and dying. Black, white, young, old, female, male, rich, poor, Southerner, or Northerner, we will all face death someday.

Sometimes the best thing to say is nothing at all. One's mere presence in the room or by the bedside is often all that is required to comfort someone. Some situations in hospice, however, require the volunteer to be more of a talker than a listener. One of these is making the initial telephone contact with the family. Usually, the volunteer coordinator (or nurse) asks the family if they would like a volunteer. If they say "yes," then the coordinator finds an appropriate volunteer and asks if he or she can take a new patient.

Once you have agreed to take a new patient, then you can call the family on the phone and introduce yourself. (Alternatively, the volunteer coordinator may introduce you to the family.) Talking to the family on the phone is often awkward. An initial phone conversation might go like this:

"Hello. May I speak to Mrs. Smith?"

(Pause) "This is she."

"My name is David Resnik. . . . I'm a volunteer from hospice."

"What? What's that?"

"Um . . . the people at hospice told me you were interested in having a volunteer to come and visit. I could do some chores, or help out with anything you might need."

"Oh." (Pause) "Oh . . . this is all so new to me. I don't really know what I am doing. The nurse came by this morning, and I said that I would like some help." (Pause) "What is it that you do?"

"It depends on what you'd like me to do. I could do some chores. I could do some shopping for you. I could come and stay with your husband in case you would like to get out of the house for a while."

"Well . . . I would like to go get my hair done this week. . . . When could you come by?"

Initial conversations seldom go this smoothly. Every time I call someone whom I don't know, I get a little bit nervous. One time I made a phone call and the caregiver/wife wanted to know if I could stay for a couple of days while she went out of town. I told her that I have my own family and really couldn't offer that kind of help. Another person thought I was trying to sell him something.

Through hospice, I have helped families in basically three ways: by doing chores, by offering companionship, or by providing respite care. Respite care (providing relief for the caregiver) is a very important (and greatly appreciated) service to the families of dying patients. Very often the primary caregiver has been taking care of the patient for a long time, sometimes for several years. She or he has spent most of her or his time with the patient, whether at home, in the hospital, or in doctors' offices. The job of a primary caregiver requires a great deal of patience, courage, and endurance.

* * *

Cody Simpson, my first hospice patient, was a seventy-four-year-old man with advanced lung cancer. He was still able to walk around and carried an oxygen tank with him wherever he went. He was tall and thin, with grayish skin and hair. Mr. Simpson once had been a very robust man, but due to his illness had wasted away. He lived in a small, one-story house with his wife, Emily. Their children and grandchildren were hundreds of miles away, and they had no other family members in the vicinity. As far as I know, they did not belong to a church. If they did, they did not receive much help from the church. So, it was just the two of them in that small house.

When I visited, Mrs. Simpson would leave the house for a little while, and Mr. Simpson and I would do chores. He was not able to lift anything heavy, but he was able to follow me around with his oxygen tank and show me what needed to be done. His main concern was to get everything ready before winter arrived. It was late August, and we had already had our first light snow. Winter held off until October thirtieth that year, when we had a major snowstorm around Halloween. Once winter arrives in Wyoming, your yard may be covered in snow until spring (mid-May).

Mr. Simpson and I cut and stacked firewood, put up the storm windows, cleaned up the yard, cleaned out the gutters, raked the leaves, and fixed the roof on the house. We also planted a few tulips for his wife. Mr. Simpson wanted to make sure that his wife would not have to do any of these chores, because he knew that he might not be around to do them. He wanted to get his affairs in order before dying.

Although it was obvious to me that Mr. Simpson knew that he was dying, he never talked about it; he talked around it. He would talk about future events, such as Christmas or spring, as if he would not be there. He would talk about how important it was that his wife would be taken care of. He was like so many people I knew in Wyoming: stoic in the face of whatever nature brings, whether it is a raging blizzard, a hailstorm, or death.

The Simpsons' house was located just outside of town, on a slight elevation above an open plain. Looking toward the west, you could see the Rocky Mountains, more than thirty-five miles away. Looking toward the east, you could see another chain of mountains, known as the Sherman Hills. Looking north and south, you could see both mountain chains extending on toward the horizon. From their house, it seemed like the whole world was an immense basin framed by distant peaks and an endless sky.

They had no trees or buildings to protect them from the wind, which blew almost constantly. The wind gathered tumbleweeds from the prairie and swept them into their yard; it ripped the shingles off their roof; it blew dust in their faces; and it made huge snowdrifts in the winter. You could feel the wind blowing even when you were inside their house. Sometimes it howled like a lonesome hound, sometimes it boomed like a jet airplane, and sometimes it screamed like an angry child. Mr. Simpson would often remark, "It's the wind that kills you." I'd remember riding my bicycle home from work after hearing about my grandmother's death and feeling like the wind was blowing right through my body.

Mr. Simpson and I did not spend much time talking about his life. We spent most of our time talking about the task at hand, the University of Wyoming football team (the Cowboys), or the weather. I did manage to learn that his family had come to Wyoming in the late 1800s and that he was a cook on a battleship during World War II. Cody continued cooking when he came home from the war. He had owned and operated a diner with Mrs. Simpson for several decades before becoming too sick to work anymore.

One week I had trouble contacting the Simpsons, who were almost always home. I soon learned of Mr. Simpson's death from the volunteer coordinator at hospice. I recall feeling some sorrow and surprise when I learned the news. Even though I expected that he would die before spring, I just never imagined it actually happening. I sent a card to Mrs. Simpson and said that I would be willing to do some chores for her, if she ever needed any help. She never contacted me. Sometimes I wonder if her tulips bloom when the snow melts.

Chapter 3

One M&M at a Time

Before becoming a hospice volunteer, I had been visiting nursing home residents. Problems regarding poor nursing home care, as well as abuse and neglect, are well-known (Glendenning and Kingston, 1999). I will not offer any solutions to these difficult economic, psychosocial, and medical issues here, but I will offer my personal observations of one method for providing patients with some hope and happiness.

One fact I discovered while visiting nursing homes is that children and dogs are very popular with the residents. Children and dogs can lead the residents to laughter and play, and give them some hope for the future. Nursing home residents look at a child and realize that life goes on, or pet a dog and know that they are loved. Over the years, I have taken my two sons, Peter and Michael, as well as our dogs, Pepper and Harry, to visit nursing homes. I have also taken large groups of children from our churches to visit nursing homes, but I would recommend bringing no more than three children at a time. Those nursing home residents who do not like children or dogs can become very agitated when children run or make noise.

* * *

The second hospice patient I met in Wyoming, George Rogers, was a sixty-nine-year-old man with lung cancer that had spread to his liver. He was living at home with his wife, Virginia Rogers. He was not able to walk around and spent much of his time in bed. He was receiving oxygen at home to help with his breathing.

Sometimes he could muster enough energy to sit up in his chair or at the table. Some friends from the Rogers' church were also helping to take care of him. The Rogerses asked for a volunteer to help out with chores around the house. They did not need any respite care, since Mrs. Rogers was receiving enough relief from members of their church.

The Rogerses were selling their house and Mrs. Rogers needed some help getting it ready to be sold. She was planning to leave Wyoming to go live with their daughter in Minnesota, after Mr. Rogers' death. The Rogerses had been planning to move to Minnesota before Mr. Rogers became terminally ill, but they decided it would be best to postpone the move because of his illness. I took down storm windows, cleaned windows and shutters, washed walls and doors, scraped paint, and picked up debris in their yard.

While I was working in their yard, I noticed that they had a lot of rocks that would be suitable homes for bugs. My son, Peter, who was four years old, was very interested in insects, spiders, and other small things that creep and crawl. I asked the Rogerses if they would allow me to bring my son with me the next time that I came to do chores. Mrs. Rogers said, "Yes, please do. . . . George would like that very much."

So I brought Peter with me the next time I visited. I told him that this yard was a good place to hunt bugs and that a man in the house would like to see him. Peter brought some jars and looked under rocks. Toward the end of our stay, Mrs. Rogers invited us to come inside the house and have a drink and a snack.

We sat down at the kitchen table with Mrs. Rogers, Mr. Rogers, and a friend from their church. She served us lemonade and soft drinks. They had a big bowl of M&Ms in the middle of the table. Peter asked if he could have some. Mrs. Rogers said, "Help yourself. . . . They're George's favorite candy." Peter and I ate some M&Ms, but Mr. Rogers did not eat any. Mrs. Rogers showed me some pictures of two young boys, about Peter's age. She told me that they were their twin grandsons who lived in Minnesota.

Mr. Rogers smiled gently as he watched Peter eating the M&Ms. He did not say a word—he just watched and smiled. Mrs. Rogers told us that George had had some rough days lately, but that he seemed better today. She said that she had not seen him this peaceful in a long time.

Peter was eating one M&M at a time. He carefully examined each one. "Do you think the blue ones taste the same as the green ones?" he asked. "I don't know; why don't you try and find out," I replied. Peter continued to eat M&Ms, and he sorted them into piles of red, orange, yellow, brown, green, and blue.

And so it went for a while. For Peter, each M&M was a new experiment, a new taste, and a new color. I also stopped eating M&Ms by the handful and started eating them one at a time. Mr. Rogers seemed to be enjoying watching Peter eat the M&Ms almost as much as Peter enjoyed eating them. I told Mrs. Rogers that we needed to go home, so that we wouldn't spoil our dinner. We thanked her for the food and drink, and we went home with several jars of bugs and a jar of M&Ms.

This was the last time that we would see Mr. and Mrs. Rogers. The next day, a hospice nurse called to tell me that Mr. Rogers had died. I sent Mrs. Rogers a note; Peter wrote his name on it as well. Mrs. Rogers soon put her house on the market and moved to Minnesota.

Mr. Rogers and Peter reminded me of an important lesson that day. When we are children, we put our whole mind and soul into each moment. We eat one M&M at a time. As we grow up, we scatter ourselves across time and space and become distracted by the future, the past, or people and events on the other side of the globe. We eat life by the handful. We worry about whether we have enough or too much, and whether other people have too much or too little. But, the truth is, all we have or will ever have is this moment, this M&M, this next breath of life. Everything else is smoke and static.

Since visiting Mr. and Mrs. Rogers, I have noticed how time seems to stand still when I visit hospice patients. Like most people in the modern world, I lead a very busy life. I have many projects, commitments, appointments, responsibilities, hobbies, and relationships. But my life becomes much more deliberate and simple when I am with hospice patients or their families. I have nothing to do but what I am asked to do, and no one to be with but whom I am with at that moment. I can take the time to appreciate autumn leaves falling from trees, the warmth of the sun on my face, the song of a sparrow, or the taste of one M&M.

Chapter 4

See the World While You Can

Soviet tyrant Joseph Stalin once said that the death of one man is a tragedy, but the death of millions is a statistic. As a hospice volunteer, I try to view death as natural, not as tragic, but also as personal and not merely as a statistic. However, some people I have known have faced unusually tragic circumstances. One of those was Karen Stallings, a nursing home resident who had been badly injured in an automobile accident. Mrs. Stallings broke her back, hips, ribs, arms, and legs in the accident. It was a miracle that she survived. Her husband of over thirty-five years, Richard Stallings, did not.

Mrs. Stallings had chronic, intractable pain. The accident had left her crippled and partially paralyzed. She had pain in her back, neck, shoulders, and legs. She also developed bedsores and shingles. Her kidneys and liver were also failing, and she had trouble eating. She was small, thin, gray, and quiet. You almost didn't know she was in the room.

Mrs. Stallings' pain was, in my judgment, very poorly managed. She had a prescription for an opioid pain medication, which she was given on a "prn" (or as-needed) basis. To get this medication, she had to ask for it. Of course, she was in no position to make demands on anyone or to assert her rights to pain relief. She would ring her call button for the nurses, but they would not come for hours on end, because they were too busy or, dare I say, didn't care. When I visited her, she would ask me to get the nurse so she could have her pain medication.

One of the principles of good pain management for severe pain is to prescribe medications on an RTC ("round-the-clock") basis, which prevents the pain from becoming worse. It is much more difficult to relieve pain that has become worse than it is to prevent pain from becoming worse. All of the hospice patients with significant pain that I have known have had pain medications prescribed on an RTC basis. Some also have had pain medications prescribed on a prn basis for "break through" pain, i.e., pain that overcomes the RTC medication regimen. Some patients I have known have refused their pain medications in order to avoid the side effects of opioid analgesics, such as nausea, constipation, sleepiness, or confusion, but all of the patients have had the *option* of taking their medication. None of them, that I know of, have had to beg for medications.

Getting back to our story, Mrs. Stallings lived in Cincinnati, Ohio, for most of her life with her husband and their pets. They never had any children, but not for lack of trying. They learned to accept their situation, and they enjoyed each other's company. They were both excellent musicians. Mr. Stallings played the piano and Mrs. Stallings played the violin. They played duets composed by Beethoven, Bach, Brahms, Mozart, and other classical musicians. They played at home, in church, and at music festivals. Although Mrs. Stallings could no longer play the violin, she was able to listen to music on her cassette player. It was one of the few things that still gave her comfort and enjoyment.

Mr. and Mrs. Stallings liked to travel, but they often found it difficult to make time to travel, due to their commitments to their jobs and community. Mr. Stallings was an insurance salesman and Mrs. Stallings was his secretary. They also belonged to the Lutheran Church, as well as civic groups, such as the Lions Club and the Salvation Army. They were planning to travel around the United States and Europe when they retired. They wanted to see the Rocky Mountains, San Francisco, Las Vegas, the Grand Canyon, New Orleans, New York, London, Paris, and Vienna.

Unfortunately, they made it only to the edge of the Rocky Mountains. Two days after leaving Ohio for a trip around the country, they were involved in a multicar pileup on Interstate 80, just outside of Laramie, Wyoming. Mrs. Stallings was treated at Ivinson Memorial Hospital in Laramie and discharged to a nursing home after two months. She found herself there, alone, in a private room, with no friends or family members within 1,000 miles. (Her younger sister had died earlier, but she had a niece living in Ohio.)

The social activities director at the nursing home asked me if I would start visiting Mrs. Stallings. She made it a point to introduce me to people who had few visitors. When I visited Mrs. Stallings, I would bring her flowers from my wife's garden and she would talk to me about her life in Ohio. She showed me pictures of her husband, her niece, and her niece's children. She also told me about her rose garden, her interest in crossword puzzles and anagrams, her enjoyment of Italian food, and her love of bridge, which she had played with her husband and other couples once a week.

She told me about all the travel plans she had made and how they had all disappeared one night. She missed her husband and wanted to be with him again. She could not understand why she didn't die with him. Mrs. Stallings told me to "see the world while you can. . . . You never know what might happen." Our visits were usually brief, because she could not endure longer ones in her condition.

I found out about Mrs. Stallings' death in the local newspaper. She had one of those short, nondescript obituaries that are printed in the section "other deaths." It said that she died after a prolonged illness, was preceded in death by her husband, and had a surviving niece in Ohio. It did not mention her plans to see the world, her love of roses or bridge, or her passion for music. In the paper, in black, white, and gray, she appeared to be another statistic. I knew better; she was a wife, a daughter, a big sister, a friend, a violinist, a secretary, a gardener, a bridge player, a traveler—a person.

Chapter 5

I Have a Dream

One of the most stressful parts of the job of primary caregiver is waiting for the end of the patient's life, not knowing when it will come. I think many people have mixed feelings about the timing of death. On the one hand, they want their loved one to continue living so that they can continue to enjoy that person's presence. On the other hand, they may want to know when their loved one will die, so that they can move on with life, and so that the loved one's suffering can end. I remember visiting one family in the hospital who had been told that their matriarch would die "any day now," and they maintained a twenty-four-hour watch in her room as she lingered for several weeks.

One woman I knew said she would wake up every couple of hours to see if her husband was still breathing. Another woman was afraid to leave the house at all because she could never forgive herself if her husband died while she was gone. Guilt is a ubiquitous ghost haunting end-of-life care. Sometimes I have to convince primary caregivers that it would probably be a good idea if they left the house for a while. Giving someone a couple of hours a week to get away from the stress of the dying process can make the difference between successful coping and a nervous breakdown.

* * *

Gloria Jones, the wife of one of the first patients I worked with when I moved to North Carolina, had been through it all. Her husband William Jones was a sixty-seven-year-old African-American man with hypertension, diabetes, and inoperable colon cancer. A series of strokes had affected his ability to walk, and he always was either in a wheelchair or his bed. He would have good days and bad days. On a good day, he would be awake and talkative. He might enjoy a glass of ice water or some cookies. He would even sing some of his favorite church hymns. On a bad day, he would be tired, cranky, nauseous, and confused.

When I visited, Mrs. Jones would leave the house to visit the hairdresser and do some shopping. When she returned, she would look calm and refreshed. We would talk a little about her husband and how she was doing before I would leave. As a man, I never really understood why some women enjoy going to the hairdresser so often. I learned from Mrs. Jones that going to the hairdresser involves much more than just getting one's hair cut; it's a way of taking time out for one's self and affirming one's self-worth. All people—but expecially caregivers—need some pampering to stay healthy and sane. I will get my hair cut when it gets too long or sloppy; some women go to the beauty parlor for different reasons, and I now respect that.

Mr. Jones had been declining steadily for the past two years, as a result of a series of strokes. Although he recovered from the strokes, his health deteriorated each time. After one of his strokes, he went home and developed the hiccups. But these were not ordinary hiccups, which go away. These were violent hiccups that lasted all day and all night for over a week and shook his whole body. The doctors gave him some medications to try to relax his muscles, but they couldn't do anything to stop these hiccups. It's amazing how something as simple as the hiccups can be so devastating. His wife was there with him through the hiccups, but this was only the beginning of their ordeal.

Mr. and Mrs. Jones had three children who lived in Virginia. Although he was born and raised in North Carolina, he had lived in Washington, DC, for many years before moving back to the Tar Heel State. Mr. Jones was very proud of his children and his grandchildren, who visited him often. He showed me pictures of his family taken in the 1970s. They all looked so happy, healthy, and beautiful. Mr. Jones told me about how he had always been there for his children: how he had taken them to football practice and baseball practice; how they had gone to Washington Redskins football games; how they loved to fish; and how they had sung together in church.

Mr. Jones was a religious man. Although I am sure that he was anxious about his impending death, he also believed that he would be going home to Jesus when he died. Mr. Jones had been a member of his church choir for many years. During his good days, we would sing some of his favorite hymns. One of them was "How Great Thou Art":

> Then sings my soul, my savior, God to thee
> How great thou art! How great thou art!

Mr. Jones also liked me to read the Bible to him. At one time he was an avid reader of newspapers, magazines, books, and the Bible, but he found it difficult to read in his final days, due to problems with his concentration and vision. Mr. Jones loved all of the Psalms, but he especially loved Psalm 91 (abbreviated here from the King James Version):

> Surely he shall deliver thee from the snare of the fowler,
> And from the noisome pestilence.
> He shall cover thee with his feathers,
> And under his wings shalt thou trust;
> His truth shall be thy shield and buckler.
> Thou shalt not be afraid for the terror by night;
> Nor for the arrow that flieth by day; . . .
> For he shall give his angels charge over thee,
> To keep thee in all thy ways.

Mr. and Mrs. Jones experienced the "terror by night" all the time. Mr. Jones still had many nights when he didn't sleep well, and he often had a difficult time getting comfortable in his chair or his bed.

Even though he had a strong religious faith, Mr. Jones still wondered a great deal about what would happen when he died and whether he would go to heaven. I have never really understood (or believed) people who say that they *know* they are going to heaven or that all their friends will be in heaven. I sometimes hear people say that a Christian should rejoice when he finds out that he is terminally ill, because he will be in heaven very soon. I think this kind of talk is intellectually and spiritually dishonest, and can be very dangerous. No human being can truly know what is on "the other side" because death is beyond our experience. The reality of death is that it is, and always will be, a profound mystery, and this, I think, is the way it should be. The great challenge of faith is to live honestly with the mystery of death and to affirm the value of life.

Getting back to our story, Mr. Jones regretted many things that he had done in his life. He wished that he had been a better husband and father. He was especially concerned about the drinking and partying he had done when he was younger. Although he had quit drinking after the strokes began, he was still worried that he had done something wrong and that he had made a fool of himself at times. He told me about how his drinking had strained his marriage to the point of almost breaking. (Mr. and Mrs. Jones were married for more than thirty years.)

I told him that no one is perfect, and that God loves us despite our mistakes and shortcomings. I also shared with him my own troubles with drinking and partying. Although I had been clean and sober for many years when I met Mr. Jones, I was able to discuss with him some regrets I had, about the bad things that I had done, and about how I had wasted some important years in my life while taking drugs or consuming alcohol. He was not able to talk to his family, friends, or his minister about the subject of drinking, so it was fortunate that I was there to hear his confession and to share mine.

Although we discussed many different topics, Mr. Jones glowed when we talked about the day that Dr. Martin Luther King Jr. gave his "I Have a Dream" speech. On August 28, 1963, Mr. Jones was working for the government in Washington, DC. He said that everyone took time off from work to go see Dr. King. Mr. Jones walked down to the Washington Mall and sat along the reflecting pool near the Lincoln Memorial. He said that he was very proud of

Dr. King and what he was doing for America. Although Mr. Jones never took part in any protests or sit-ins, he supported the civil rights movement. He adored Dr. King, President John F. Kennedy, and his brother Robert Kennedy, and he mourned when each of these leaders was assassinated. Dr. King's vision (available at <http://www.mecca.org/~crights/dream.html>) still conveys tremendous courage and wisdom:

> I have a dream that one day even the state of Mississippi,
> A desert state, sweltering with the heat of injustice and oppression,
> Will be transformed into an oasis of freedom and justice.
> I have a dream that my four children will one day live in a nation
> Where they will not be judged by the color of their skin
> But by the content of their character.

Mr. Jones had been to Mississippi and had been judged by the color of his skin. In the late 1950s, he took a business trip to Mississippi by himself in a car. He was filling his gas tank at night when several white men assaulted him. They were planning to lynch him. Fortunately, the police broke up the incident and Mr. Jones escaped with his life. He drove back to North Carolina as fast as he could. He told me that there were places that colored people just did not go to in those days, out of fear of racial violence. He also told me what it was like to have been excluded from restaurants, schools, and hospitals, to have to use a separate rest room, and to have to sit in the back of the bus. I realized then how much the country had changed in forty years, but also how far it still has to go.

Before I met Mr. Jones, the "I Have a Dream" speech was something I had studied in history books. I had seen it on television many times. I had discussed the injustice of racism in college and university classes, both as a student and as a teacher. I had discussed the arguments for and against affirmative action ad nauseum. None of this had as much of an impact on me as talking with Mr. Jones. In my relationship with him, I learned how racism had harmed one black man, and how it might be possible to overcome it.

At some point, Mr. Jones suddenly underwent a precipitous decline. When I first met Mr. Jones, he had been able to walk with a walker. Then he became too weak to walk, but he was still able to sit up in a chair. In the last few weeks of his life, he found it very difficult to be comfortable in his chair, and he spent most of his time in bed. He was very agitated in his bed and had difficulty sleeping. His wife said that he scared her one night because he woke her up talking to people who were not in the room. Mr. Jones claimed that he was talking to his parents, who had died many years ago. Other hospice patients and families that I have known have reported similar experiences. Although I have found their accounts hard to believe, I have never dissuaded them. I have simply listened and acknowledged their beliefs and concerns.

Mr. Jones's children and grandchildren came to visit him sometime around Christmas. He made a brief rally for the visit, and then he died two days later. I attended his funeral, which was a very beautiful and moving ceremony, with many testimonials about his life and much singing, weeping, and laughing. Mrs. Jones decided to move out of their house and near her children in Virginia. The last time I saw her was at a yard sale she organized to prepare for moving. I bought a couple of items, including a music book and a Washington Redskins cup.

Chapter 6

I Can Fix It

Most of the patients and family members that I have visited go through a stage of grieving known as denial. Denial is the first stage of responding to a major loss or disappointment. One simply pretends that the loss has not happened or will not happen. Most people move through this stage and go through the other stages of grief—anger, bargaining, depression, and, finally, acceptance. No set timetable exists for moving through these different stages. Each person who suffers a loss must come to terms with the loss in his or her own way.

Unfortunately, some people get stuck in the denial stage and never move beyond it. People have many different ways of denying the reality of death. Many patients and their families use their religious beliefs to deny death, declaring that "God will perform a miracle." I have seen family members in the intensive care unit of the hospital tell a doctor that he should not take their brain-dead father off life support because that would prevent God from working a miracle. Personally, I believe that if God is going to work a miracle, He won't let a piece of fancy technology get in his way. If He can help Moses part the Red Sea, then He doesn't need a respirator to bring a patient back to life.

In my opinion, this idea that God will perform a miracle, like the idea that anyone could know that they will go to heaven, is intellectually and spiritually dishonest. It turns God into a servant catering to human desires. Just as nothing guarantees we will get into heaven (if there is a heaven), nothing guarantees that a miracle will happen. If we are honest with ourselves, we will realize that a miracle probably won't happen. A miracle could happen, of course, but why should we be so arrogant as to expect that by asking for a miracle we can make it happen?

Honesty demands that we understand the powers of modern medical technology as well as its limitations. Doctors have the power to keep people who would have died in a different era alive for years. Respirators, ventilators, heart-lung machines, defibrillators, pacemakers, bypass surgery, organ transplants, and dialysis machines are wonderful medical inventions and innovations that can be used to save lives. But we must use these tools wisely, and refrain from using them if they will only prolong human suffering or needlessly forestall death.

Sometimes medical treatments are inappropriate or futile. A couple of years ago, a team of doctors at Duke University spent over 5 million dollars trying to keep a patient alive over a thirty-four-day period and almost created a worldwide shortage in rare clotting factors (Winslow, 2001). Finally, the doctors and the family agreed that the treatment wasn't working, and they let the patient die. We once had a patient in hospice with end-stage leukemia who needed weekly blood transfusions to stay alive. As he became more and more ill, he needed transfusions twice a week; he had to decide when he would stop the transfusions and allow himself to die. As did this man, all dying patients must eventually decide to "let go" of the world and move on.

But some patients just won't let go. Some patients hang onto life with incredible tenacity and stubbornness, denying the reality of death until their last gasp. Buck Johnson was one of those patients. He was a seventy-nine-year-old man with lung cancer. He lived with his wife, Betty, who had chronic back pain from several compressed disks in her spine. In addition to caring for Mr. Johnson, Mrs. Johnson also had to care for her ninety-seven-year-old mother, who lived next door. Mrs. Johnson's mother was actually in better health than either Mr. or Mrs. Johnson.

As a result of his cancer, Mr. Johnson had virtually no function in his left lung. A hospice nurse said that the lung was not moving air. His doctor prescribed some medications to help with his pain and breathing, as well as oxygen. Mr. Johnson denied that he had cancer. He said that he was "going to beat this thing." When the nurse asked him why he thought he was having trouble breathing, he said that he had some allergies, but that he would get over them. Mrs. Johnson was worried that Mr. Johnson was not accepting his disease, but she also realized that she could not do much to change his mind. I never confronted Mr. Johnson about his cancer, but I encouraged him to take his medication as directed, and to take care of himself and ensure his own safety.

Mr. Johnson was a handyman, a jack-of-all-trades, and an entrepreneur. The son of a sharecropper, Mr. Johnson worked in the tobacco fields of North Carolina as a boy. He did not complete high school, but he earned his high school equivalency diploma years later. He was self-educated and self-made. He had worked on tobacco farms, on dairy farms, and in orange groves. He had owned and operated a sawmill, an automobile repair shop, and a general store. He had sold insurance and was a certified financial planner. He had worked as an appliance repairman and as a carpenter. He had been a commercial truck driver for many years and owned some used trucks. He also had driven cars, tow trucks, motorcycles, tractors, bulldozers, buses, and backhoes. He had operated drills, chainsaws, table saws, lathes, electric welders, and computers. He wanted to fly an airplane, but he never got around to it. Mr. Johnson had a workshop next to his house. Prior to his illness, he had enjoyed working with wood and tinkering with old televisions, lawn mowers, and appliances.

Mr. Johnson had medications to treat his pain, but he tried to avoid taking them. He had an oxygen tank for his breathing, but he tried to avoid using it. He rationed his medications and oxygen and used them only when his pain became unbearable or his breathing became almost impossible. He did not want to become dependent on the medications or the oxygen. In his mind, if he needed less medication or oxygen, this meant that he was getting better. If he needed more, this meant that he was getting sicker.

Mr. Johnson was no longer a safe driver. His doctors told him that he needed to use his oxygen tank to drive, but he insisted that he didn't need it. He said that he could get enough air if he adjusted the air conditioner to blow in his face, and he continued to drive, using this "remedy." One day he lost consciousness while trying to turn out of a parking lot and had a minor collision. The accident injured his left shoulder. Finally, he stopped driving.

Mrs. Johnson needed some help buying groceries and picking up medications. She could drive, but she could not stay on her feet long enough to walk around a store, because her back hurt too much. Each week, Mrs. Johnson told me her grocery list over the phone, and I bought the items that they needed. When I dropped off the groceries, I also visited for a little while.

One day when I visited, Mr. Johnson showed me the deeds to some land that he owned in another county, which he had bought as an investment for himself and his family. The land was not cleared or well marked. Mr. Johnson told me that people who owned land next to his were building a trailer park on his land. He said that he needed to do something to prevent the "squatters" from stealing his land. This upset him very much, and he talked about it whenever I visited, until he died. He seemed much more concerned about this hypothetical threat to his property than the real threat to his life.

Mr. Johnson lived much longer than his doctor thought that he would. I think I visited him for about seven months. Each time I visited, he would tell me more stories about his home remedies or his savvy solutions for domestic, political, and financial problems. He could fix almost anything, but he couldn't fix his cancer.

When the inevitable happened, Mrs. Johnson invited me to her house for one more visit. I brought my son Michael with me, who was three years old at the time. Peter and Michael had visited the Johnsons a few times, and the Johnsons enjoyed their company. Michael noticed that the chair in which Mr. Johnson usually sat was empty. He asked, "Where is Mr. Johnson?" I looked into Mrs. Johnson's eyes, which were beginning to tear up. She then replied, calmly and peacefully, "He's not here anymore, darlin'. . . . He's gone to heaven."

Chapter 7

Piggly Wiggly Has the Best Service

Many of the patients I have visited begin to detach from the world as they prepare to die. They let go of the world by withdrawing from life. They become introverted and reserved and prefer solitude and quiet during their final days. Frank Wilson was not one of those patients. Mr. Wilson loved telling stories and being around all types of people. He was interested in current events on television and continued to read the newspaper and do crossword puzzles. He was quick-witted and had a keen sense of humor. He was fully engaged in life until the day he died. He was a warm, charming, and gentle person, who could captivate his audience when he spoke. His voice was strong but soothing, like fresh-brewed coffee.

Mr. Wilson was an eighty-four-year-old Caucasian male with lung cancer, emphysema, hypertension, and congestive heart failure. His doctor discovered the cancer when Mr. Wilson was hospitalized with pneumonia. Because the cancer was inoperable, Mr. Wilson decided to forgo chemotherapy in favor of hospice care. Mr. Wilson had an oxygen tank to assist his breathing. He was weak from his heart and lung conditions, as well as from a stroke, from which he had not fully recovered. He could still walk with a walker, but he was unable to drive or take care of his daily needs. Mr. Wilson was not a large man: he was of medium height with a slight build. He was thin even before he developed cancer.

When I began visiting Mr. Wilson, I discovered that two people in the house were dying. Mr. Wilson's wife, Lisa Wilson, had advanced Alzheimer's disease and dementia. She was no longer able to communicate meaningfully or feed, dress, or bathe herself. She could still swallow and walk, but she spent most of her time in bed. When she tried to talk, she sang out like a chorus of birds. She would do this whenever she was excited. It sounded like "Aahhyeeeaaahyeeeiiiiilllaaallaaayyeeeiiii . . ." Mr. Wilson would say, "There she goes, singing again."

Mrs. Wilson was a friendly person who smiled often, especially when someone entered the room. Although her mind was wasting away, her body was still in very good condition. Mr. Wilson would joke that "If you put the two of us together, my mind and her body, you'd have one healthy person."

Mr. Wilson loved his wife dearly, despite her profound illness. He said that he still thought that she was "the most beautiful woman in the world," and that she was his "best friend." He loved to hold hands with her and snuggle with her in their bed. He was concerned about her well-being and always wanted to know how she was doing. They were married for sixty years.

Because the Wilsons could not take care of themselves, they needed a lot of help in order to avoid going to a nursing home. Their three children, Margaret Piner, Carol Watson, and Robert Wilson, pooled their resources to allow their parents to continue living at home. They hired an African-American woman, Clara Hendricks, to stay with their parents. Ms. Hendricks cooked, cleaned, and shopped. She also helped the Wilsons bathe, dress, and eat. Hospice nurses also provided care for the Wilsons. The children took turns visiting their parents.

Margaret Piner was a nurse who was familiar with hospice and palliative care. Margaret followed her parents' care closely and did her best to prevent them from dying in a hospital or nursing home. Before her parents became seriously ill, she had a discussion with them about how they would like to be cared for at the end of life. Both of her parents wanted to die with dignity and comfort, at home. They did not want high-tech, curative medicine. They both signed health care power of attorney documents, naming Margaret Piner as their health care agent (someone who can make a medical decision for someone else). They also signed living wills. Mr. Wilson also wrote a one-page note describing his religious beliefs and moral values.

My role on the hospice team was to provide companionship for Mr. Wilson, who missed his wife's company. Even though she was still present with him, he could no longer talk to her. When he did, she would sing unintelligibly, and he would stop. Mr. Wilson needed an audience for his stories. Everyone else had already heard his stories many times, but I was a fresh face, willing to listen. After I got to know Mr. Wilson, I also noticed that he was telling the same stories over and over again, but I didn't mind. Mr. Wilson told stories about his family members, his friends, his employment, his education, and his childhood and youth.

One of the stories I remember was about Mr. Wilson's college days. Mr. Wilson attended East Carolina Women's College, which has since become East Carolina University. When Mr. Wilson attended East Carolina, 300 women and only ten men were enrolled in the college. Mr. Wilson said that during his senior year, he dated Deborah Barnes, the "prettiest girl in the whole school." Because he didn't consider himself to be very attractive, he was amazed that "someone like that would date a guy like me."

Mr. Wilson didn't date his gorgeous girlfriend again after they graduated from East Carolina. One year after graduation, Mr. Wilson had married his wife, Lisa, and Ms. Barnes was still single. Ms. Barnes came by to visit Mr. and Mrs. Wilson one evening, which made Mrs. Wilson very jealous.

Another story that he liked to tell was about his son, Robert. Mr. Wilson said that when Robert was about four years old, he saw Mr. Wilson shaving in the bathroom. Robert said, "Dad, when I grow up, I want to be big, just like you." Mr. Wilson found this to be amusing, since he was not a large man. He said it took his son ten years to discover that his father was not very big.

When I heard Mr. Wilson's story about his son, I asked him if he would like my son Michael, who was then four years old, to visit. Mr. Wilson said, "Of course; I'd love to meet him," so I brought Michael with me for most of our visits from then on.

What Michael remembers about visiting Mr. Wilson was going to Piggly Wiggly, a grocery store. Mr. Wilson still liked to get out of the house to shop. I would drive him around in his old Buick. He would tell me which way to go—he preferred to take the route with less traffic and more scenery—and we would stop at several stores. As we drove, Mr. Wilson would tell me stories about different places around town, as well as his opinions about poorly kept houses or overbuilt areas.

What Mr. Wilson liked the most about Piggly Wiggly was its service. "They have the best service," he would say. Good service was very important to Mr. Wilson. He enjoyed talking to the cashiers, salespeople, and managers of the stores, and he was on a first-name basis with all of them. He preferred to go to small, locally owned stores, instead of huge chains such as Wal-Mart, Walgreen's, or Food Lion. I sometimes think about Mr. Wilson when I go to a store that does not have good service, and I wonder why I go there. Am I interested only in convenience or economy?

Although Mr. Wilson valued good service, he also liked hunting for bargains. Each week he would look for specials and coupons in the newspapers. He would cut these out and bring them with him on our trips, along with some cash and a shopping list. When he was at the store, he would buy fruit that was a little too ripe, but still good, and bread that was out-of-date, but not stale. He bought store brands, not name brands, and he took note of the price per unit and price per ounce. Mr. Wilson, like many people of his generation, learned about spending money during the Great Depression. He was not stingy, but he did know how to spend his money responsibly and wisely. His attitude toward money stands in sharp contrast to today's credit-crazy society.

In the stores, I pushed the cart, Mr. Wilson walked alongside me, and Michael walked in front. Mr. Wilson would ask Michael to help him find items he needed. When we got to the checkout line, he would tell the cashiers, "I've got my two helpers with me today."

Mr. Wilson seemed to know almost everyone in town. Everywhere we went, he would say hello to someone or tell me that he knew someone living in a particular house. He met many people through his work. For more than forty years, he purchased tobacco from farmers for Philip Morris. Greenville was the center of tobacco farming in eastern Carolina. Tobacco farmers from all across the eastern part of the state would bring their harvests to the tobacco market. During harvesttime, the smell of fresh tobacco would permeate the whole town. Although I do not like the smell of burning tobacco, fresh tobacco has a rich, fresh, and almost medicinal smell.

Mr. Wilson also met many people through Little League baseball. He was a big fan of Little League. He coached teams and went to many games. He also raised money to construct baseball fields around Greenville. The year before I met Mr. Wilson, Greenville's all-star team went to the Little League World Series. Mr. Wilson also belonged to the Jaycees, which raised money for projects in town.

One day, Mr. Wilson showed me his piano and his harmonica collection. I asked him if he could play anything. He did not have enough breath to play the harmonica, but he was able to play some Scott Joplin rags on the piano and some church songs. He sang a few bars of "Amazing Grace," before running out of breath. Mr. Wilson allowed Michael to play his piano. He told me that the piano used to belong to his mother, who was very musical. She taught all of the children how to sing and play music. Mr. Wilson told me that during the Depression, his family had to sell a piano that they owned, but that once the difficult times had passed, they bought a new one.

Mr. Wilson's health declined rapidly during his last few weeks of life. He developed pneumonia and was hospitalized. When I visited him in the hospital, he was disoriented and confused. He was discharged back to his home after a few days in the hospital, but he got pneumonia again a couple of weeks later and died at home, with his family at his side.

Mr. Wilson's children asked me to be a pallbearer at his funeral. They said that I was one of his best friends during his last five months of life. I was honored to serve in this capacity. Mr. Wilson's children held two services at their church, a regular service and a special service for Mrs. Wilson, who could not sit through the regular service. At her special service, which preceded the regular service, Mrs. Wilson saw Mr. Wilson in his coffin and began singing. I think she understood that he was leaving. After the regular service, the procession of vehicles drove out to the graveyard, where Mr. Wilson was laid to rest. At the graveside, his son, Robert Wilson, played "Amazing Grace" on one of Mr. Wilson's harmonicas.

Michael, who is now eight years old, still remembers Mr. Wilson. He says that he misses going to Piggly Wiggly with him. I still remember Mr. Wilson too, and I will always think of him when I hear "Amazing Grace."

Chapter 8

Give Yourself Some Living Room

As a teacher volunteering for hospice, I have only once had a patient who was also a teacher. Darrell Miller was a teacher, but not in the usual sense. He did not teach elementary school, high school, or college or university students. He taught truck drivers how to handle their rigs and the basics of driver safety.

Mr. Miller was a seventy-year-old man with chronic, obstructive pulmonary disease and congestive heart failure. His breathing was very poor, and his heart was weak. He had oxygen and many medications to treat his pulmonary and cardiovascular problems. I visited Mr. Miller once a week for a couple of months to provide him with some company and give his wife a break from caring for him.

Mr. Miller was an independent truck driver for more than thirty years. He drove through every state in the continental United States at least twice. He never once had an accident that was his fault. He loved his wife and children dearly, but he also enjoyed being on the road, seeing different sights and meeting different people.

When he finished his career as a truck driver, he settled down and became a teacher. He was a driver's education instructor and taught a course to help truck drivers prepare for their commercial license exam, which he helped the state of North Carolina design. Mr. Miller was interested in my work, and he wanted to know what it was like to teach at the college and university level. He asked me questions about philosophy and ethics. We also talked about his life on the road, what different parts of the United States were like, and Elvis Presley's music.

A piece of advice that Mr. Miller gave me still sticks in my mind: "Give yourself some living room." This rule is easy to understand, but rarely followed in today's hurried society. I wish more drivers on the interstate highways and crowded cities would practice what Mr. Miller preached.

What Mr. Miller meant by his slogan is that you should make sure you leave plenty of space between your vehicle and the other vehicles on the road. You need enough space in front of you, so that you can stop in time if the car in front of you slows down; you need enough space behind you, so that the car behind you won't crash into you if you slow down; and you need enough space on both sides, so that you can move out of the way to avoid a potential accident. The rule is very simple: you want to avoid being boxed in when driving. You need room to maneuver, room to live.

When I drive on our crowded highways and streets, I try to give myself some living room, but it seems that someone is always filling it up. On the highway, I usually leave plenty of space between my vehicle and the one in front of it. When I do this, aggressive drivers take advantage of the space and squeeze in, in front of me. I let off of the gas to make more space, but then someone else fills it up. I try to avoid driving side by side with other vehicles, but I often find myself crowded in. And so it goes.

A corollary of Mr. Miller's rule is "Lay off the brake." If you are using the brake too much, then you are probably not giving yourself enough room when you drive, you are driving too fast, or both. I have seen people violate both of Mr. Miller's rules on the road. A driver in a hurry will rush in front of someone and then tailgate the car in front of him. To avoid hitting the car, the driver must put on his brakes, which will cause the car behind him to put on his brakes, and the dominoes will fall. Eventually, traffic far behind the tailgater will slow down or even stop from the accumulated braking. All of this could have been avoided if the drivers had practiced Mr. Miller's rules. Traffic flows much more smoothly when people are cooperating on the road instead of competing.

Why do people do this? Why are so many people in such a big hurry on the road that they would risk dying to get where they are going? Why do people have to race with one another on the road?

Why is road rage a common phenomenon in American cities, such as Los Angeles?

Mr. Miller's explanation is that these problems are symptoms of a society that has lost its way on the road and in life. People want to get somewhere so fast that they forget how to treat one another along the way. They forget about safety. They forget about civility. They forget about honor. They forget about fairness. They even forget how to relax and have fun.

Mr. Miller's solutions were simple and straightforward. Slow down. Be careful. Be civil. Be honorable. Be fair. Stop and smell the roses. Give yourself some room.

These are lessons that I have heard many times before, but they became real for me when they came from the mouth of Mr. Miller. When he told them to me, I was slowing down and I was listening. Whenever I drive now, I remember to give myself some living room.

Chapter 9

Plant a Garden

After several years as a hospice volunteer, I had learned many lessons about death and dying from the patients that I worked with, but none were more important than the lessons I learned from my wife's cousin, Kristi Kunkel, who died from pneumonia at age thirty-two. She endured more pain than I can imagine, yet she was a very positive person, who displayed tremendous courage, faith, and hope. Although she was not a hospice patient, she embodied the hospice philosophy of spiritual growth at the end of life. Although she was slowly dying, she celebrated life.

Kristi had been seriously ill for over a decade, with an autoimmune disease known as lupus. Her death took place piece by piece, as her own immune cells attacked different parts of her body. Among other symptoms, the disease affected her joints, causing rheumatoid arthritis. Kristi found it difficult to walk or do anything with her hands, such as playing the piano or typing. The disease also eroded her bones and teeth. She had an operation to replace her jawbone, and she eventually lost her teeth. She had frequent bouts of pancreatitis and gastrointestinal problems. Because she found it so difficult to eat or keep her food down, she weighed less than ninety pounds (at 5' 4" tall) just before she died. She was hospitalized several times each year. A team of doctors and her faithful husband, Norman Kunkel, cared for her.

Kristi's health problems began at an early age. As a young child, she suffered from migraine headaches and allergies. As she continued to grow, she developed curvature of the spine, which caused pain and discomfort. While in college, Kristi had an operation to correct her back problem. The surgeons straightened out her spine with metal rods. Kristi's medical purgatory became much worse after the surgery. She had an allergic reaction to the metal rods, which had to be replaced. The operation also stretched and realigned her internal organs, triggering her first episode of pancreatitis. It is possible that her reaction to the surgery triggered her lupus, although we do not know this for a fact.

Kristi suffered through many different health problems before her doctors finally determined that lupus was the underlying cause. Lupus can be a difficult condition to diagnose; no definitive tests for this illness exist. It took her doctors a long time to reach a diagnosis because she did not have any of the characteristic markers of the disease, such as facial blemishes. It seemed all we would ever hear about her was that she was sick again, or in the hospital again. Kristi told me that she had lupus a couple of years before she died. She had been frustrated when her doctors didn't know what was wrong with her, and she was somewhat relieved to at least know what was killing her.

I met Kristi when I was in graduate school at the University of North Carolina–Chapel Hill, and she was an undergraduate student at North Carolina State. Kristi's parents, Ron and Barbara Hardee, invited my wife and me over to visit Kristi and her younger sister. The Hardees were (and still are) big NC State Wolfpack fans. They were all wearing red and white (NC State's colors) and I was wearing light blue (UNC's color). They teased me, just a little bit, about my loyalty to the UNC Tar Heels.

Kristi was a very bright and talented woman. She majored in biochemistry and had a strong science background, but she also had an appreciation for literature, science fiction, philosophy, film, art, and music. She had planned to go to law school one day to practice environmental law, but she was not able to fulfill that dream. She was a passionate gardener and collector of pottery, sculpture, and glass. Although she was a very serious and diligent person, she also had a keen sense of humor and a sharp wit. Like her father, she enjoyed practical jokes.

Susan and Kristi had a strong relationship, one that has survived Kristi's death. They had many common interests, such as gardening, herbal medicine, and antiques. Their personalities also meshed. They had been pen pals for many years, and Susan asked Kristi to be a bridesmaid in our wedding. After Kristi died, Susan planted a garden in honor of Kristi in our backyard. The garden is shaped like a heart. It has some of Kristi's favorite flowers and herbs, with a dwarf Japanese maple tree in the middle and a small statue of an angel on the right side. Sometimes when Susan is in our backyard she talks to Kristi. I have also sent my thoughts and prayers to Kristi, wherever she may be now. And, at times, it seems as if she answers back.

Kristi met Norman when they were both students at NC State. Norman, who was studying engineering, was devoted to Kristi. He knew that Kristi had serious medical problems when he met her, but this did not prevent him from falling in love with her or standing by her in sickness and in health. They both enjoyed sailing, skiing, and waterskiing together. After their wedding, they made their home in Davidson, North Carolina, where Norman worked as a nuclear engineer. They had two dogs, but no children. Kristi had wanted to have a baby, but she could not due to her illness. She had a job as a biochemist for a while, but had to give that up when her illness worsened.

We did not see much of Kristi when we lived in Wyoming. We made the 1,800-mile journey between Wyoming and North Carolina one or two times a year to visit family during the holidays or at other significant times, such as weddings or funerals. We also saw family members when they traveled west. One January, we met Kristi, Norm, and Norm's parents in Colorado, where they were skiing. Kristi was not able to ski with them, but she was able to appreciate the Rocky Mountains in winter.

When we moved back to North Carolina in 1998, Kristi's physical health had declined dramatically but her spiritual health had improved. When we saw her, she would talk about her problems, but she also asked us about our lives. Some people, when they become ill or debilitated, spend all their time talking about or worrying about their own health. Kristi was not one of these people. Kristi had relied on her faith in God to help her cope with her sickness and suffering. She saw the beauty in nature and in people as evidence of God's handiwork. She was seriously ill, but she was not desperate. She had lost much of her health and vigor, but she was grateful for what she had left.

I remember visiting Kristi and Norm in Davidson in the spring of 1999. The dogwood trees were blooming; the birds were singing; everything was warm, green, and lush. Kristi took us on a tour of the plant life around her house. She and Norman had built a variety of gardens, including a water garden. She had many different flowers, herbs, and shrubs. She cherished each plant as if it were a newborn child, and invited us to behold its wonders. During my visit, I felt inspired to write a poem for Kristi:

SPRING REBIRTH

The sparrows proclaim spring's rebirth
From winter's dark and tragic mirth.
The flowers explode with radiant hues—
Tulip red, dogwood white, and iris blue.

Daffodils dance a goldfinch tune
And cardinals conduct azaleas in bloom.
The squirrels court among the trees
And butterflies flitter on the breeze.

The rabbits sneak a morning bite
While fawns recline in the sunlight.
The new leaves weave a canopy
Above this lush and fertile bed.

Warm showers bring nourishment
To the legacy of the dead.
Seasons transform grief and sorrow
Through love's cultivation:

Tears become rain, death becomes hope,
And despair, jubilation.

Kristi loved the poem and shared it with her friends. She encouraged me to write more poems, and I was inspired. I had written a great deal of poetry when I was in high school and college, but once I started pursuing my academic career, I invested most of my creative energies in scholarly writing. I continued writing poems and sending them to Kristi until she died. One of the poems I wrote for her was about morning:

EARLY IN THE MORNING

Listen to the songbirds sing
Early in the morning.
Hear the world rise up and ring
Early in the morning.

The daybreak is a gift from God
The dawn of love's redeeming.
Watch the little children play
And join them in their dreaming.

The honeysuckle fills the air
Early in the morning.
Its soft sweet scent's beyond compare
Early in the morning.

The flowers that grow among the fields
Show God's love everywhere.
Plant your garden every day
And say a morning prayer.

Feel the breeze upon your face
Early in the morning.
Behold the daylight's saving grace
Early in the morning.

The evening storm has cleared away
And left its healing water

A bright new sun has now shown us
The glory of the Father.

The last time I saw Kristi was when she and Norman stayed at our house, while they were visiting Kristi's sister, in Washington, North Carolina. Beth, who was now married to Jack Wilder, had given birth to a baby girl, Mary Grace Wilder, a few months earlier. Kristi stayed at our house so that she could get some rest and visit with us as well. Kristi loved Mary Grace as if she were her own daughter. Kristi knew that she would never have children, but she wanted to watch Mary Grace grow, play, and live.

I can remember it taking Kristi a long time to get out of bed in the morning, because she was so weak and stiff, and in so much pain. We talked about her illness, about pain and symptom management, about doctors, about religion, and about death. While watching Kristi deteriorate over the years, I wondered from time to time how her disease would progress and when or how she would die. Although I did not consider her to be terminally ill, I did not expect her to live for a long time. I would think to myself, "How much more can she endure?" every time I heard about her illness flaring up again. Kristi shared with me her own thoughts about death and about how difficult it was to keep going on, in such pain. She said that she was very tired and felt like giving up, but that she would go on.

Kristi died a few months after that visit. I was very sad, but I also knew that her suffering had ended. More than anything, I was upset that she had had such a difficult life. It didn't seem fair that someone so wonderful would have such an awful disease. But, who said life was fair? Kristi did not complain about her lot in life. Indeed, she considered life to be a blessing. She was not bitter about her condition or jealous of healthy people. She did the best that she could with what life had given her.

Even though Kristi had been very sick for many years, her death came as a surprise. Most of her family members, myself included, were in various stages of denial. Although we didn't think she would be cured of her illness, we imagined that she would continue her struggle with it. As it turned out, she was much more aware of her own mortality than most of us. She had talked to Norman about end-of-life decisions. She also told him that he had her blessing to marry someone else after she died. In her journal, she had talked about where she wanted to be buried, and she had selected some music to be played at her funeral.

Today, I like to imagine that Kristi is watching over us, like a guardian angel. Sometimes I talk to Kristi when I am near her garden in our backyard. I mow carefully around the rocky border, I look at the statue of the angel, and I smell the scent of thyme and oregano. And sometimes I think I hear her voice telling me to plant and garden, and to write poetry.

Chapter 10

I Need to Go to Church

Becoming a hospice volunteer has helped me learn to trust that still small voice inside of me. We all have different names for that voice: some call it God; some call it Allah; some call it the Holy Spirit; some call it wisdom; and some call it conscience. But whatever we call that voice, we all sometimes look to it for moral guidance.

An experience I had with this voice taught me to pay attention to it. One Friday, the volunteer coordinator asked me if I would take a new patient. I said that I would be available. The volunteer coordinator gave me some background on the patient. Mr. Brodie was a sixty-five-year-old male with kidney cancer. He had had a devastating stroke two months before that rendered him comatose. Mr. Brodie had been in the hospital for more than three months, but his wife finally decided that it was time to let him go, and she opted for hospice care. She stopped his dialysis treatments, although she did not request that his feeding tube be removed.

I telephoned the patient's wife, Wanda Brodie, and she asked if I could visit on Sunday morning so that she could go to church. I initially said that I couldn't come by on Sunday because I had my own family and church obligations that morning, but that I could come by later in the week. She said that would be fine, but I could tell by her voice that she really wanted me to visit on Sunday.

I started having second thoughts about saying no to Mrs. Brodie's request for Sunday. I thought to myself, *What would God want me to do? Would he want me in church with my family on Sunday morning or would he want me staying with a dying man so that his wife could go to church?* I turned this over a few times but decided, again, that it would be enough to visit later in the week. I asked my wife about it, and she said she would like for me to be in church with our family, but that she would certainly understand if I had hospice work to do. Either way, I would be doing God's work.

Later that night, as I was saying a few prayers before bedtime, I heard a voice telling me, in no uncertain terms, to go to visit the Brodies on Sunday. I felt an anxious and urgent feeling inside me. I *had* to listen to that voice. So I listened, and I obeyed. The next morning I called up Mrs. Brodie and told her that I would come by on Sunday. She was very excited and thanked me.

On Sunday, I drove out to the Brodies' home and arrived at 9 a.m. Mrs. Brodie invited me inside. She wanted me to stay past lunchtime, because her church was about a thirty-minute drive away. I said that would be fine. She showed me around their house—a double-wide mobile home—and showed me where Mr. Brodie was staying. She said that he was very quiet and that I wouldn't need to do anything for him. She showed me the hospice phone number to call in case of an emergency.

I had never seen anyone still alive yet so close to death. Mr. Brodie's dark-brown skin had an ashen tone to it. His breathing was long, slow, and weak. He did not move in his bed. His hands and face were also noticeably swollen. I noticed that he had a feeding tube, which was unusual for hospice. Most people who choose hospice care also refuse artificial hydration and nutrition, but this is not a requirement for being admitted to a hospice. Although artificial nutrition and hydration can extend life in dying patients, they can also exacerbate suffering by causing swelling, breathing difficulties, and regurgitation of food. In any case, it did not look like Mr. Brodie would live for a long period of time, with or without his feeding tube.

Mrs. Brodie drove to church. I caught up on some reading, watched some television, and checked on Mr. Brodie every once in a while to make sure that he was still breathing.

When she returned, it seemed like a tremendous weight had been lifted off her shoulders. She wore a nice smile and was joyful. She told me that she had not been to church since Mr. Brodie had been in the hospital, and that she really missed her friends there, the singing, and the worship. She asked if she could do anything for me, and I said, "No, thank you"; it was my Christian duty to help. She understood, but she still sent me home with some cupcakes for my two boys. Before I left, I told her I could come back on Tuesday morning to visit.

It was cold, rainy, and wet when I arrived on Tuesday morning. A blue car that I did not recognize was parked outside the Brodies' trailer. When I went to the door, a nurse from hospice opened it and told me that Mr. Brodie had died just a short time before my arrival. The nurse invited me inside the home. I greeted Mrs. Brodie. I gave her a hug and told her I was sorry. One of her neighbors was also with her. The hospice nurse told me that she tried to call but couldn't reach me before I left my home. I said that I didn't mind making the trip and that I was glad to be there. We talked for a little while, and then a black hearse pulled up next to the blue car.

Mrs. Brodie, the nurse, and the neighbor went out to talk to the funeral home director, who was standing outside with a black umbrella. I took this occasion to say good-bye to Mr. Brodie. I knelt down right next to his bed and said a few prayers. When I had finished, I left the room, went outside, and said good-bye to Mrs. Brodie and the nurse.

As I drove down the muddy road, I felt distressed. I did not expect to see a dead man that day, but these things happen in hospice. I thought about what would have happened if I had not listened to that voice, and then I knew that I had been at the right place at the right time and with the right words. A feeling of calm and a sense of purpose came over me as I realized that I had done my part, however small it might have been, to help this family in a time of transition and sorrow.

Chapter 11

I Knew You Were Okay When I Saw You Pull Up in a Ford Truck

Eastern North Carolina has seen many hurricanes over the years. They have brought devastating winds, spawned furious tornados, pulled along tremendous storm surges, whipped up erosive tides, and killed many people. Floyd was a relatively mild hurricane when compared to powerful storms such as Hazel (1954), David (1979), or Fran (1996). What Floyd lacked in raw force he more than made up for in water. Floyd dumped more than a foot of rain in places that were already saturated from two previous hurricanes. The ensuing flood did more economic damage to North Carolina than any other natural disaster. The waters flooded houses, buildings, factories, farms, and airports, and washed away bridges, roads, cars, crops, animals, and people. Some people were killed, thousands lost their jobs, thousands more lost everything that they had, and many others were surrounded by water for days. Even those people who were not directly affected suffered indirect effects, such as the loss of electricity, clean water, food, or gasoline. It has been almost six years since Floyd hit, but many people have not yet recovered financially or emotionally from the hurricane. Some Floyd survivors become very agitated and fearful whenever there is a long, hard rain or a flash flood.

Floyd did not inflict significant damage on my house or family. As did everyone else, we lost a few trees as well as electric power and clean water, but we were able to resume our lives with relative ease. The worst thing that happened to us is that we found ourselves inundated by water snakes, some of them poisonous. None of the hospice patients I knew lost their lives as a direct result of Floyd, either, but the hurricane created considerable havoc for hospice patients and workers. Rescue workers removed elderly, disabled, and sick people from their homes and brought them to shelters. Some hospice patients went to a hospital or other facility, but most remained in their homes. Hospice nurses made heroic efforts to visit patients and to make sure that they still had contact with the outside world. The hospice patient that I was visiting at that time was well cared for.

If nature had her way, most of eastern North Carolina would be a swamp. Human beings have temporarily changed the course of the land by draining wet areas, digging ditches, and moving dirt. For a few weeks in the fall of 1999, nature reclaimed her dominion. When the Tar River flooded, it spread out across the flat eastern Carolina countryside like milk spilled on a table. The river covered the entire Pitt County Airport, which is about five miles north of the river. Many of the houses damaged by the flood had only a few feet of water in them, but this was enough to ruin them. A couple of feet in the elevation of a building could make the difference between safety and destruction.

The water was contaminated with everything that the flood had carried in its wake, including sewage, garbage, and animal carcasses. The water had a foul, rotting odor, like vinegar and honey mixed with dead opossums.

* * *

About six months after Floyd, in March 2000, I was assigned a hospice family, the Worthingtons, who were still struggling with the aftermath. The family lived in an area of Pitt County that had been under water for a few weeks. The Worthingtons' house barely escaped Floyd's wrath. A two-foot-high brick foundation supports their house. Because the water came up about six inches below the top of the foundation, their house was spared, although they had to deal with mold, mildew, fire ants, snakes, and the stench of the floodwater. However, for about ten days they were isolated in their house, which was surrounded by water. They did not want to leave their property, so rescue and hospice workers brought them food, water, and medicine.

As I drove out to see the Worthingtons, I could see many houses that Floyd had ruined. Most were deserted, with stacks of furniture, clothing, and possessions piled in front of them. I pulled my green 1994 Ford Ranger into their driveway and parked around the back of their white house, next to a storage shed. I knocked on the back door, just below the "WARNING: OXYGEN IN USE" sign. Mary Worthington greeted me with a smile that she just managed to pull across her vexed face.

"Hi. I'm David Resnik, the hospice volunteer," I said.

"Hi. I'm Mary Worthington." (She paused, then gave a fuller smile.) "I knew you were okay when I saw you pull up in a Ford truck," she said.

I had never really thought of my truck as a welcome sight, but I accepted her comment, and said, "I like it. . . . It's reliable."

I then noticed that they had a white Ford truck parked around the back of the house. "Won't you come on in," she said.

As I got to know Mrs. Worthington, I could tell that she really needed people whom she considered to be "okay." She had been through much in the past few years, and she did not need anything else to worry about. Her husband, Chuck Worthington, was a sixty-eight-year-old man who had been very ill with obstructive pulmonary disease and congestive heart failure. Both of these diseases are chronic and progressive. The lifestyle he had led when he was younger—he was a smoker, a hearty eater, and poor exerciser—had taken its toll on his health. He also had hypertension and diabetes. Mr. Worthington would become fatigued and short of breath very quickly: he found it difficult to walk from his bed to his chair or even to carry on a conversation. His hands and feet were swollen, even though he was taking medications to prevent him from retaining water.

Mr. Worthington came from a farming family. He inherited his house and land from his father, who inherited them from his father, who inherited them from his father, back all the way to the Colonial era. The dirt road in front of their house was named after their family. The house looked like it had been built in different stages, as if each generation had added its own addition or renovation. The entire house had been raised the crucial two feet off the ground after Hurricane Fran. The property was so old that they had no deeds as proof of ownership. Instead, the family had a charter from King George III of England. That's how long they had lived in Pitt County.

Mr. Worthington had followed the family farming tradition, but he strayed from it after his father died at age fifty-two. When he was younger, he had grown tobacco, cotton, corn, soybeans, watermelons, and tomatoes. But he got tired of farming (he couldn't take the heartache and frustration of being a small-time farmer anymore, he said), so he went to college and worked for a bank. He had sold some of his land and bought stocks, which he followed every day on the financial channel on cable television. He still owned about 100 acres of land, which he leased to farmers.

Mr. Worthington took early retirement, due to his declining health. Mrs. Worthington had been taking care of him for more than four years. She had been driving him to the doctor and the hospital, supervising his medications, and, when he got worse, helping him to dress and bathe. During the flood, she made sure that he had enough oxygen and medication. After the flood, she also began managing their finances and tending to the family's business.

Mrs. Worthington worked as an office assistant in a busy medical practice. She performed the administrative tasks that no medical practice can do without, such as greeting patients, giving them forms to fill out, answering the phone, and dealing with insurance companies. When Mr. Worthington retired, Mrs. Worthington continued working, but on a part-time basis so that she could take care of him and deal with her own health problems.

Mrs. Worthington had fibromyalgia, a mysterious illness that many doctors regard as psychosomatic, perhaps because they do not understand its physical basis. Doctors who do not believe that the disease is real refer to it as a "syndrome." Those who believe that the disease is real think that it may be caused by damage to the nerves that relay pain signals to the brain or those that process pain signals in the brain. This type of pain is known as neuropathic pain. For example, doctors now know that "phantom limb pain," in which patients experience pain from an amputated limb, results from damage to the body's pain sensation system.

Of course, these academic disputes make little difference to the patients who must deal with the disease. Mrs. Worthington had pain in her jaw, face, neck, shoulders, and back. She also suffered from anxiety, depression, and fatigue. She took medications to help control her pain, anxiety, and depression. She also used swimming and massage therapy to manage her disease.

When I visited, Mrs. Worthington would leave the house to go swimming and to receive some massage therapy. When she returned, she would look relaxed and at ease. We would spend some time talking about Mr. Worthington and her disease before I would leave. I believed that her disease was real, and I offered her sympathy and support. We talked about living with chronic pain and the idea that it might not be cured, but that it could be managed. In Wyoming, I knew chronic pain patients and the doctors and nurses who helped them. I joined a pain coalition formed by the wife of a man with chronic, neuropathic pain. When I talked to Mrs. Worthington, I was reminded of Mumu's chronic pain. I wondered again whether Mumu might still be alive if she and her doctor had sought to manage, rather than cure, her pain.

I did not get to know Mr. Worthington very well during our visits. He spent most of his time in bed. When he was in his chair, he could not talk for very long, because he would lose his breath. Like most hospice patients that I have known, he loved music. They had an old piano in their living room, which I played for him. They had several songbooks and hymnals. I played mostly Christian hymns, such as "Amazing Grace," "What a Friend We Have in Jesus," and "Joyful, Joyful, We Adore Thee." Mr. Worthington, a veteran of the Korean War, also enjoyed patriotic music, such as "America, the Beautiful." One of his favorite songs was "There's a Land That Is Fairer Than Day," also known as "Sweet By and By":

> In the sweet by and by,
> We shall meet on that beautiful shore.

Mrs. Worthington also enjoyed the music. She had played the piano when she was younger, but she hadn't played in years. She decided to have it tuned again so that I could play.

Mr. Worthington died in his bed one night after I paid a visit. He succumbed to pneumonia and stopped breathing. I wrote Mrs. Worthington a condolence note, and I received a nice note in return. She invited me to bring my two boys out to her house for a visit. She had grandchildren, but they lived far away. Peter hunted for bugs around their house and Michael tagged along. Mrs. Worthington did not seem to be terribly distraught that Mr. Worthington had died. In fact, she admitted that she was somewhat relieved. He (and she) suffered greatly during his last six months of life. He struggled to stand, to walk, to talk, and to breathe. She struggled to take care of him, to comfort him, and finally to let him go to that "sweet by and by."

Mrs. Worthington said that she was very saddened by her loss, but she would learn to deal with it, much in the way that she had learned to deal with her chronic pain. Through hospice, I have learned that grief can be like that. You might not ever cure it, but you can learn to live with it.

Chapter 12

You Don't Know All the Bad Things I've Done

Prejudices take many forms. The most obvious and destructive ones are those that we have laws against—i.e., prejudice based on race, religion, gender, or ethnicity. Although we have made much progress in dealing with these types of prejudices, Dr. Martin Luther King Jr.'s dream remains just that—a dream. More subtle forms of prejudice can also cause considerable suffering and injustice to society. People who are short, fat, or ugly are likely to earn less money in our society than people who are tall, thin, and beautiful (Stossel, 2005; Teachman et al., 2003). Superficial though it may be, people often are judged according to how they look or speak.

Prejudice based on one's locality and culture is another significant issue in the United States. For many people, the Civil War never completely ended. Prejudices based on old animosities exist on both sides of the Mason-Dixon Line. Some Northerners call Southerners "hicks," "rednecks," and "grits," while some Southerners refer to Northerners as "damn Yankees," "carpetbaggers," and "ugly Northerners." Southerners often are depicted in popular books, movies, and television series as ignorant, provincial, and racist. Northerners, especially New Yorkers, are portrayed as loud, angry, and bossy. Although it seems the media has slandered Southerners more than Northerners, both groups have had to face stigmas and biases.

My family moved to Chapel Hill, North Carolina, in 1967, when I was five years old. Because my parents were not from the

South, and I had spent the first five years of my life out of the South, I never developed a southern accent. As a white boy with a plain accent and strange name growing up in the South, I learned about prejudice against Northerners. People would hear me speak and ask in a threatening way, "Where are you from?" and "What kind of a name is that?" With the name "David Resnik" and an accent that was definitely not southern, I looked and sounded like a "damn Yankee." Worse yet, I might even be a Jew.

Since my youth, many Northerners have migrated to the South, and Southerners are becoming accustomed to (and perhaps tolerant of) northern people. Today, people who hear my name are more likely to ask, "Oh, are you related to so-and-so Resnik?" than they are likely to ask, "What kind of a name is that?"

My wife, Susan, who grew up in Wilmington, North Carolina, has a mild southern accent. Her speech is clear and charming. It is not the slow, illiterate drawl one hears on *The Beverly Hillbillies* or *The Dukes of Hazzard*. Even so, when we were living in Wyoming, some people made fun of her accent. Although their behavior amounted to little more than teasing, they were still treating her differently based on the way she talked. She felt like they were pegging her as a dumb southern girl.

One of the hospice patients I knew, Patrick O'Brien, was a victim of prejudice against Northerners. Mr. O'Brien spent most of his life in upstate New York. He and his wife, Kate, had moved south a few years after he retired to escape the frigid northern winters and to be near their daughter, Candy Langley, who was a nurse working in Greenville, North Carolina. Mr. O'Brien was Irish Catholic and spoke with an Irish accent. He loved New York's professional athletic teams: the Yankees, the Knicks, the Rangers, and the Jets.

Mr. O'Brien was not in good health when he moved to North Carolina: he had heart failure, hypertension, and diabetes. His health became much worse after being attacked by his neighbor, Hilda Taylor. Mr. O'Brien's home was next to Ms. Taylor's home in a trailer park. Ms. Taylor spent a lot of time tending to her flowers, and she did not like Mr. O'Brien mowing near them. She had yelled at him several times about mowing near her flowers. One day he had just finished mowing near her flowers and he was beginning to weed his tomatoes. He was bent down on the ground with his back turned to her, when she took a shovel and hit him in the middle of the back. He cried out in pain and fell forward on his stomach. Then she hit him again on the back and face.

The attack paralyzed Mr. O'Brien from the middle of the back down to his feet. He spent a couple of months recovering in the hospital before he was sent home. He had contacted the county sheriff about the incident when it happened. Ms. Taylor told the sheriff that Mr. O'Brien attacked her first and that she was just trying to defend herself. It was her word against his. The prosecutor told Mr. O'Brien that he would not press charges against Ms. Taylor, because a jury would not believe Mr. O'Brien's side of the story because he was a Northerner. Who would a jury of Southerners believe: a pushy, Irish-Catholic man from the North or a polite, Pitt County resident and fellow Southerner? Mr. O'Brien also faced a roadblock from personal injury attorneys, who told him that they would not bring a lawsuit against Ms. Taylor because she did not have much money.

Mr. O'Brien still had a great deal of physical and emotional pain from the attack when I met him. He had pain in his back, shoulders, neck, and abdomen. He had difficulty breathing and eating. He was tall (6' 3") and very thin (130 pounds). His face was taut, with a grayish undertone. His hair was white and thinning. He was very weak, but he was also restless; he would frequently pull himself up in bed or move from side to side. He had a portrait of Jesus on one wall and a crucifix on the other.

Mrs. O'Brien was staying with him, but she could not do very much to help him because she had dementia and hearing difficulties. Whenever I spoke to her, I could never get much more out of her than "okay." Their daughter lived in the same trailer park. When she came home from work, she prepared meals for them and took care of other chores. Some tension existed between Mrs. O'Brien and her daughter; they argued whenever I saw them together. I think that Ms. Langley was frustrated by her mother's dementia and hearing difficulties.

My visits with Mr. O'Brien provided him with some companionship. We talked about his life in upstate New York, the long winters, his family, and his work (he had been a salesman). We talked about his religious faith and contemporary moral issues, such as capital punishment. He talked openly about dying and admitted that he was afraid.

He liked to recite the Lord's Prayer:

> Our father, who art in heaven,
> Hallowed be thy name;
> Thy kingdom come,
> Thy will be done,
> On earth as it is in heaven.
> Give us this day
> Our daily bread
> And forgive us our sins
> As we forgive those who sin against us.
> And lead us not into temptation
> But deliver us from evil.
> For thine is the kingdom,
> The power and the glory,
> Forever.
> Amen.

One day he said to me, "I don't think I'm going to the good place."

"What do you mean?" I said.

"You know; I might be going down 'there.'"

"I don't think so. . . . You've lived a good life, haven't you?"

"You don't know all of the bad things that I've done."

"I've done some bad things too. We all do bad things. I believe that God can forgive us if we confess our sins."

"But you don't know what I've done."

"What have you done? Have you harmed anyone badly?"

"No."

"Have you broken any laws?"

"No. I haven't been nice to people. I'm not a nice person."

"You seem perfectly nice to me."

"But you don't know me well."

"Well, I'm not the one to judge. All I can do is pray for you."

The conversation continued from there. He expressed his worries about what would happen to him after death, and I listened and tried to reassure him. We talked about how he had been involved in the church and civic groups for many years and about some of the other good things he had done, such as being a father, a husband, a brother, and a friend. After a while, he was too weak to talk anymore, so we stopped.

Because he could not talk for very long during our visits, I asked Mr. O'Brien if he would like me to bring my electronic keyboard, so that I could play some music. He said that he would love to hear some music. From that point on, I played music for him during my visits. Mr. O'Brien loved hymns, as well as some popular songs from the radio, theater, and movies. Some of his favorites were "When Irish Eyes Are Smiling," "Ole Man River," "Galveston," "Swing Low, Sweet Chariot," "Raindrops Keep Falling on My Head," "Somewhere Over the Rainbow," "Send in the Clowns," and "I Can't Help Falling in Love with You." He would close his eyes and listen when I played, and sometimes he would drift off to sleep, peacefully.

Mr. O'Brien died a couple of days after one such visit. Of all the patients that I have known, he seemed the most fearful of death and dying. Even though he was a religious man, he had doubts, regrets, and misgivings. On earth, an imperfect legal system denied him justice. I hope that, in death, he found justice and forgiveness.

Chapter 13

He Was a Helluva Ballplayer

Almost all of the hospice patients whom I have known were aware that they were dying, at some level. A few talked openly about death, while some talked around it or denied it. A couple of patients that I knew could no longer talk at all when I met them, but I am fairly certain that they knew about their impending death before losing the ability to communicate. One of the patients that I knew, Rudy Nowitzski, was alert, conscious, honest, open, and talkative, but he was totally unaware that he was dying. He contradicted all of the stereotypes that one learns about grief, despair, and religious hope in dying patients. His awareness was focused entirely on the present moment, with little care or concern for the future.

Mr. Nowitzski was an eighty-year-old man with lung cancer that had spread to his brain. The tumor in his brain affected his ability to process information about recent events or think about future ones, although it did not affect his memory of the distant past or his ability to meaningfully interact with people. He was very good at talking about what was going on right in front of him, but when the conversation would require him to go beyond the present, he would become confused and would confabulate. For example, he was aware that Hurricane Isabel existed, but he did not know whether it was coming or had already come. If I asked him about something in the immediate past and he didn't know the answer, he would say, "I'm not quite sure. . . . I can't remember anything anymore."

He also had elaborate delusions concerning the weather, activities around the house, his finances, and other matters. He told me one time that a chandelier in his home had a speaker inside of it and that it could talk to him and control things in the room. Whenever the weather changed, he would tell me that "it must be the mountain acting up again." Several times he told me a story about lightning coming off the mountain and knocking him out of bed and injuring his knee. (The nearest mountain was more than 200 miles away and lightning never struck inside the house.) He said that his son had sold his house for him for about $11,000. (His son did sell his house, but for much more than $11,000.)

Despite these problems with his memory and cognition, he was able to carry on a conversation and to make minor decisions. He could talk about sports, the weather, his family, or his past. He asked me questions about my work, health, and family. He was able to watch television and listen to music. He was good company, as long as you stayed within his limits and tolerated his mistakes and delusions, which was not too difficult for me to do.

Although Mr. Nowitzski had terminal cancer, in other regards his health was excellent. He was not in any significant pain or discomfort. He was able to eat, talk, sit up, and walk (with a walker). He had no difficulty breathing, and he was a very pleasant person. When I met him, I did not think he was sick enough to be a hospice patient, and I thought they might discharge him. (Sometimes patients are discharged from hospice if they are not sick enough to qualify for hospice care.) However, his nurse said that he would remain in hospice, because he had a brain tumor. His health could rapidly decline at any time.

Mr. Nowitzski's lung cancer, which developed slowly, was discovered by accident. His doctors found the cancer when he was admitted to the hospital for pneumonia and mental status changes. Because of his advanced age and the extent of his cancer, his family decided to not make him go through surgery or chemotherapy. He was referred to a local hospice, even though he did not know what that meant.

Mr. Nowitzski lived with his oldest son, Rudy Jr., his daughter-in-law, Sharon (who was a nurse), and their nineteen-year-old twin daughters, Stacy and Stephanie, who were both enrolled in college and living at home. Mr. Nowitzski's wife died from cancer several years before. When his wife died, he wrote a living will and named Rudy Nowitzski Jr. as his health care power of attorney. Rudy Sr. also completed a legal document giving general power of attorney to Rudy Jr., so that Rudy Jr. could take care of his finances, which included selling Mr. Nowitzski's house. Between the four of them and the hospice nurses, Mr. Nowitzski was well cared for.

My role on the hospice team was to provide Mr. Nowitzski with companionship. On the first day I went to visit him, I met him and Sharon Nowitzski. I told him that I was a hospice volunteer, and I explained to him that hospice works with patients who are terminally ill. This did not register with him, so I did not push the topic any further. As we continued our conversation, I could tell that he was having some problems responding appropriately to what I said. We talked for a while longer, and he started telling me some bizarre stories.

As I was leaving, Sharon walked me out to my truck and told me about Mr. Nowitzski's disease and mental problems. She told me that they had decided to not tell him that he was terminally ill, because he would not be able to understand this, and talking about it would only make him upset and confused. She said that he knew he was sick and that he was being taken care of, but that's about all he could handle. I apologized for mentioning the nature of his illness to him. She told me not to worry about that, since my remark went "right over his head."

In an earlier era, it was common to not tell people that they were terminally ill. Some cultures still accept this practice and believe that even talking about death is bad luck. I normally believe in complete honesty with patients and their families, because this promotes effective decision making, acceptance of death and dying, and spiritual growth. Although I would not force a person who insists on denying the truth to confront it, I believe that one should not hide or varnish the truth. One should speak the truth, openly, candidly, and lovingly.

In Mr. Nowitzski's case, however, I was more concerned with helping him enjoy his final days than telling him the truth about his situation, because he was not capable of understanding his condition or making decisions about it. I believe that talking to him candidly about his health and trying to help him work through issues related to death and dying would have made him upset and confused, and would not have helped him have a peaceful death. We did, in fact, talk about death, dying, and artificial life support when we were watching a television show that examined the subject, and he even told me that he did not want to be kept alive artificially. However, we never talked about specific details of his diagnosis or prognosis. He knew that he was not well, that he had been in the hospital, that he was well cared for, and that he was not in any significant pain. That's all he needed to know.

Mr. Nowitzski's favorite subject was sports. He had played baseball, football, and basketball while attending high school in New Jersey. He was a star baseball player at Penn State University, and he also played baseball while serving in the army during World War II. After the war, he played minor-league baseball for a while, but he gave that up and started working for the United States Postal Service, where he was employed for more than thirty-five years. He continued to follow sports throughout his life and attended many of the Yankees' baseball games while living in New Jersey. He also supported Little League and youth baseball as a coach and patron. He moved to Greensboro, North Carolina, with his wife in 1973.

Because I am also a dedicated baseball fan, I enjoyed listening to Mr. Nowitzski's stories about the great baseball stars that he saw play, including Joe DiMaggio, Mickey Mantle, Duke Snider, Willie Mays, Jackie Robinson, Bob Feller, Yogi Berra, Pee Wee Reese, Whitey Ford, Don Larsen, Sandy Koufax, Roger Maris, Ted Williams, and many others. Even though he could not remember what he ate for lunch, he could remember everything you wanted to know about the 1956 World Series or Mickey Mantle's career. ("The Mick" was his favorite ballplayer.) We watched baseball games on television, including some games from the 2003 Major League playoffs and World Series. When we talked about some of the great baseball players of times past, Mr. Nowitzski would often remark, "He was a helluva ballplayer."

We talked about going to see the Kinston Indians play minor-league baseball. I offered to take him to a game, but I never got the chance. His son ended up taking him to the last baseball game he would ever see in person. Mr. Nowitzski told me all about the game the next time I saw him, and added, "I wish you were there."

Mr. Nowitzski also loved to watch movies. We spent some time watching movies on cable television and on videotape. Watching television was a good activity for him, because it was something he could focus on without becoming confused. We could have a conversation about what was happening on the television, even though we might not be able to talk about current events reported in the newspaper. He enjoyed action movies and comedies more than complex dramas, because these genres were easier for him to follow. For every movie we watched, he would say, "I think I've seen this one before."

Mr. Nowitzski also enjoyed baseball movies, including *Bull Durham* (one of my favorites) and *Pride of the Yankees,* which is the story of Lou Gehrig—another one of Mr. Nowitzski's favorite ballplayers—and his battle with the disease (amyotrophic lateral sclerosis or ALS) that now bears his name. Gehrig set the record for most consecutive games played at 2,130, a record that stood for fifty-six years until Cal Ripken Jr. broke it on September 6, 1995. Gehrig hit 493 home runs, drove in 1,995 runs, and had a .340 life-time batting average. He was modest, kind, dependable, and hard-working. He ended his consecutive-game streak on April 30, 1939, after getting no hits in four at bats, which dropped his batting average to .143. His performance had declined the previous year, but he did not know why. Two months after his streak ended, he was diagnosed with ALS, and he retired from the game. The Yankees honored Gehrig during a break in a doubleheader with the Washington Senators on July 4, 1939. Gehrig gave a famous speech that left many in the crowd of more than 60,000 in tears. He acknowledged that he had had a bad break but that he still considered himself "the luckiest man on the face of the earth" (available at <http://www.historychannel.com/speeches/archive/speech_109.html>).

Mr. Nowitzski also considered himself to be very lucky. He knew that he was ill, but he was very grateful that he had people who were taking care of him. He often remarked that his son and daughter-in-law were "taking care of everything. . . . I don't have to worry about anything." Sharon Nowitzski told me that he was also very grateful for my visits and always looked forward to them. He wasn't exactly sure when I had visited him or when I would be visiting him next, but he knew that I was there. He would tell people proudly, "I have a friend coming to visit me today."

I visited Mr. Nowitzski almost every week from May to December 2003. After a couple of months of visiting him, I started bringing my electronic keyboard and I played some songs for him and his daughter-in-law. He enjoyed religious hymns as well as some popular songs, such as "Memory," "Someday My Prince Will Come," "When You Wish Upon a Star," "Stardust," and "Moon River." After Thanksgiving, I played some Christmas music, both religious and secular songs.

By the third week of December, I had visited him for more than six months, and I was beginning to wonder when he would pass away. He seemed to be healthy enough to continue living at least another year or two. Would I continue visiting him for another year? Waiting for the finality of death can be difficult, even for someone who is only a hospice volunteer. During what was to be my last visit, I noticed that he had a slight cough and that he seemed a bit tired. He did not appear to have the flu, pneumonia, or even a bad cold. I found out a couple of days later that he had died in his sleep the night after I visited. The family held the funeral in Greensboro, where he had lived much of his life. I wrote them a condolence note and told them how much I had enjoyed spending time with Mr. Nowitzski. They wrote me a thank-you note and told me how much Mr. Nowitzski had looked forward to my visits. I will always think of him when I watch the Yankees or the Kinston Indians play. He was a helluva ballplayer.

Chapter 14

Euthanasia

"Euthanasia" comes from the Greek words "eu," which means "good" or "well," and "thanatos," which means death. How could death be "good"? One might say that a good death is simply one that is not bad, i.e., a death that is free from pain, suffering, or indignity. In modern times, "euthanasia" has become synonymous with intentionally killing an animal or a person in order to bring about a good or merciful death. Although hospice tries to help dying patients and their families to have a good dying experience, it does not endorse or condone intentionally killing people or helping them to commit suicide.

In the time that I have been a hospice volunteer, no patient or family member that I have known has ever requested euthanasia or assistance in a suicide. I think this is due, in large part, to the fact that hospice does a very good job of controlling pain, mitigating suffering, and helping people achieve acceptance and hope through the dying process.

However, it also has been my experience that many patients and family members who have chosen hospice still think about or talk about other options. I think many dying patients who express an interest in euthanasia or assisted suicide want to know that these options are available to them, even if they choose not to pursue them.

Personally, I believe that patients who are competent and terminally ill should have the right to choose euthanasia or suicide. Because death is such a personal and private experience, we should have the right to make choices about how we die, as long as these choices do not harm other people. If it's my life to live, it is also my life to relinquish. However, I also realize that significant social, political, and economic problems with legalizing euthanasia or assisted suicide exist. It might be very difficult to prevent abuses, such as taking the life of someone who is not terminally ill or taking the life of someone who has not made a voluntary choice to die. Thus, although I think euthanasia or assisted suicide may be morally acceptable in some cases, I do not think that these practices should be legal. For further discussion of these issues, see *Intending Death: The Ethics of Assisted Suicide and Euthanasia* (Beauchamp, 1996) and *Physician-Assisted Suicide: What Are the Issues?* (Kopelman and De Ville, 2001).

* * *

Our culture has invented sanitized expressions for discussing performing euthanasia on animals. When I was a child, we had a family dog, who had gotten very old and sick. We took her to the vet to have her "put to sleep." We also had an old horse "put down" and a cat "laid to rest." I remember being very sad when these animals died, much sadder, at least in the short run, than when some family members died.

For many people, the death of a pet is their first significant experience with grief. Probably everyone remembers when their cat, dog, fish, bird, hamster, or horse died. As we mature, many of us are taught that grieving for the loss of a pet is childish and immature. How could the loss of a pet compare to the loss of a parent, a child, or a spouse?

I once felt this way, but I no longer do. I have come to learn, through my work with hospice, that all grief is the same, whether one is grieving the loss of a pet, a car, a college experience, a job, or a person. In grief, we come to terms with the undeniable fact that everything in life changes, and that we cannot hold on to anything forever. We must eventually learn to let go of everything and everyone that we will ever know.

Before Susan and I had any children, we owned a silver-gray miniature poodle named Pepper. He was, in many ways, our first child. We got Pepper after we had been married a couple of

And the antelope roam the plains
And the aspen shimmer and sigh
And the wildflowers bloom and shine
And the streams are fresh and cold
And the little dogs smell the wind
And never grow tired and old.

So good-bye for now, old friend.
I'll see you again some day.
I'll meet you in the Wyoming spring:
I know you will find your way.

For about a week after Pepper died, I seemed to be able to see him out of the corner of my eye. I would think that I saw him, look, and he would not be there. Susan told me that she experienced the same phenomenon. Were we seeing a ghost? Was the image just a fantasy created by our minds to deal with the grief? Or were our eyes playing tricks on us by expecting to see something that wasn't there? We will probably never know.

I have tried to understand why my sorrow for Pepper's death was so intense and, in some ways, cathartic. I have come to believe that the reason my feelings were so intense is that when I grieved for Pepper, I also grieved for all of my other losses. Pepper symbolized, for me, something that was gone forever. When I thought of him, I also thought of different times in my life that were now over—the first years of my marriage with Susan, completing my doctorate, life in Wyoming, and Peter and Michael's early childhoods. Pepper lived through all of these times. When he died, it was as if a part of my life died with him. And that sadness, I believe, is at the root of all grief: whenever we grieve for anyone, or anything, we are ultimately grieving for ourselves. Pepper's death represented the death of everyone that I will ever know, including me.

I also think that my sorrow was so intense because it was so private. The death of a human being is a very public event. After a prolonged illness, accident, or sudden event, a declaration of death occurs, followed by disposition of the body through embalming, cremation, or some other socially sanctioned process. Next, a memorial service or funeral is held, perhaps accompanied by a visitation and a graveside service. An obituary appears in one or perhaps several papers. People offer condolence cards, letters, and flowers. Often, an estate is settled, which usually involves lawyers, judges, courts, and banks. Other rules govern the mourning period. For example, people are expected to wear black or somber colors, and widows or widowers are expected to wait an appropriate length of time before remarrying. To help the survivors control themselves during these public events as well as the mourning period, a doctor may prescribe sedatives or antidepressants. All of this public activity is important, to be sure, but it can sanitize, sedate, and cloak the raw, uncontrollable, deeply felt emotions that occur in private grieving.

So, it is not childish to experience profound sadness at the death of a pet. Grief for the loss of a pet is not second-rate grief. It is real and important, and deserves recognition and respect. An animal may not be a human being, but it is something that we love, receive love from, care for, cherish, hold, learn from, and finally, must let go.

I included this chapter in a book about hospice volunteering because Pepper's death evoked many of the same feelings I experienced when people that I knew died. Understanding my attachment to this animal and my sadness at his death helped me to get a clearer perspective on the loss of other people in my life. Although he was *only* a pet, for me he symbolized the joy of life and the challenge of death.

Bibliography

Beauchamp, Tom (ed.) (1996). *Intending Death: The Ethics of Assisted Suicide and Euthanasia.* Upper Saddle River, NJ: Prentice-Hall.
Bereseford, Larry (1993). *The Hospice Handbook: A Complete Guide.* Boston: Little and Brown.
Byock, Ira (1997). *Dying Well.* New York: Riverhead Books.
Federal Rules of Evidence (2001-2002 Edition) (2002). St. Paul, MN: West Publishing.
Glendenning, Frank and Kingston, Paul (eds.) (1999). *Elder Abuse and Neglect in Residential Settings: Different National Backgrounds and Similar Responses.* Binghamton, NY: The Haworth Press.
Kelley, Patricia and Callahan, Maggie (1992). *Final Gifts.* New York: Poseidon Press.
Kopelman, Loretta and De Ville, Kenneth (eds.) (2001). *Physician-Assisted Suicide: What Are the Issues?* Dordrecht, the Netherlands: Kluwer Academic Publishers.
Kübler-Ross, Elisabeth (1997). *On Death and Dying.* New York: Scribner.
Kuhl, David (2002). *What Dying People Want.* New York: Doubleday.
Nuland, Sherwin (1994). *How We Die.* New York: Alfred A. Knopf.
Singh, Kathleen (1998). *The Grace in Dying: How We Are Transformed Spiritually As We Die.* San Francisco: Harper.
Stossel, John (2005). "The ugly truth about beauty." Available at: <http://www.ABCnews.com>.
Teachman, Bethany; Gapinski, Kathrine; Brownell, Kelly; Rawlins, Melissa; and Jeyaram, Subathra (2003). Demonstrations of Implicit Anti-Fat Bias: The Impact of Providing Causal Information and Evoking Empathy. *Health Psychology* 22(1): 68-78.
Webb, Marilyn (1997). *The Good Death.* New York: Bantam Books.
Winslow, Ron (2001). "Intensive care: One patient 34 days in the hospital, a bill for $5.2 million." *The Wall Street Journal,* August 2, p. A1.

Index

Active listening, 3-5
Alcohol use, regret over, 24
"Amazing Grace," 35, 36
Anger, stage of grief, *xii*
Animals, euthanizing, 72-78
Assisted suicide, 71-72

Baseball movies, 69
Baseball players, 68, 69
Bull Durham, 69

Caregivers, stories of
  Brodie, Wanda, 49-51
  Jones, Gloria, 21-26
Children
  author's, visiting hospice patients, 33-34, 58
  as caregivers, 61, 66-67
  helpful to nursing home residents, 13
  patients and their, 32
Clergy, listening and, 4

Death
  fear of, 62-63
  as a public event, 77-78
Dementia, 4, 65-66
Denial, stage of grief, *xii,* 27
Discharge, from hospice care, 66
Dog(s)
  helpful to nursing home residents, 13
  Pepper, story of, 72-77
Do-not-resuscitate (DNR) order, *xii*
Dying declarations, rule, *ix*
Dying Well, 2

"Early in the Morning," poem, 45-46
End-of-life decisions, 47
Euthanasia
  and animals, 72-78
  and humans, 71-72

Federal Rules of Evidence, ix
Fibromyalgia, 56-57
Final Gifts, 2
Floyd, hurricane, 53-54

Garden, as memorial, 43
Gehrig, Lou, 69
"Give yourself some living room," advice, 38
"Good Bye, Old Friend," poem, 76-77
Good Death, The, 2
Grace in Dying, The, 2
Grief, 77
  anger, stage of, *xii*
  denial, stage of, *xii,* 27
Guilt, and primary caregivers, 21

Hearsay, law on, *ix*
Heaven, 23-24
Hospice
  approach, 1-2
  discharge from, 66
  emergence of, 1
  training, author's own, 3
How We Die, 2
Hurricane Floyd, 53-54
Hymns, patients listening to, 57, 63, 70

"I Have a Dream" speech, 24-25
Illness, not telling patient gravity of, 67-68
Internal voice, listening to, 49-50

Joint Commission on the Accreditation of Healthcare Organizations, 2

King Jr., Dr. Marin Luther, 24-25

"Lay off the brake," advice, 38
"Let go," inability to, 28-30
Listening, active, 3-5
Living will, 32
Lord's Prayer, 62
"Luckiest man on the face of the earth, the" speech, 69
Lupus, 41

Medical treatment, inappropriate, 28
Medicare, 2
M&Ms, story of, 14-15
Moral guidance, 49
Multidisciplinary approach, hospice, 2
Music, patients enjoying author's, 57, 63, 70

National Hospice and Palliative Care Organization, 2
Neurotic pain, 57

Pain medication, round-the-clock, 17-19
Pallbearer, author as, 35
Patients, stories of
   Johnson, Buck, 28-30
   Mr. Jones, 22-26
   Kunkel, Kristi, 41-47
   Miller, Darrell, 37-39

Patients, stories of *(continued)*
   Nowitzski, Rudy, 65-70
   O'Brien, Patrick, 60-63
   Rogers, George, 13-15
   Simpson, Cody, 9-11
   Stallings, Karen, 17-19
   Wilson, Frank, 31-36
   Worthington, Chuck, 55-58
Patriotic music, patients enjoying, 57
Pepper the dog, story of, 72-77
Phantom limb pain, 57
Phone call, introductory, 8
Piggly Wiggly visits, story of, 33-34
Piner, Margaret, nurse, 32
Poems, author's
   "Early in the Morning," 45-46
   "Good Bye, Old Friend," 76-77
   "Spring Rebirth," 44
Prejudism, 25, 59-61
Pride of the Yankees, 69
Primary caregiver, children as, 61, 66-67
Primary caregiver, stories of
   Brodie, Wanda, 49-51
   Jones, Gloria, 21-26
Psalm 91, 23
Public event, death as a, 77-78
"Put down," animal, 75

Racial segregation, 25
Religious beliefs, patients and, 23
Resnik, Muriel, *x-xii*
Respite care, 8-9
Ripken Jr., Cal, 69
Round-the-clock pain medication, 17-19

Segregation, racial, 25
Sports, 68-69
"Spring Rebirth," poem, 44
Stress, and the primary caregiver, 21

Teacher
    the dying as a, x
    patient, Darrell Miller, 37-39
Television, watching with patients, 69
"Terror by night," 23

Web sites
    "I Have a Dream" speech, 25
    "Luckiest man on the face of the
        earth, the" speech, 69
    National Hospice and Palliative
        Care Organization, 2
What Dying People Want, 2

Order a copy of this book with this form or online at:
http://www.haworthpress.com/store/product.asp?sku=5259

DYING DECLARATIONS
Notes from a Hospice Volunteer

_____ in hardbound at $24.95 (ISBN-13: 978-0-7890-2544-9; ISBN-10: 0-7890-2544-2)

_____ in softbound at $14.95 (ISBN-13: 978-0-7890-2545-6; ISBN-10: 0-7890-2545-0)

Or order online and use special offer code HEC25 in the shopping cart.

COST OF BOOKS_____	☐ **BILL ME LATER:** (Bill-me option is good on US/Canada/Mexico orders only; not good to jobbers, wholesalers, or subscription agencies.)
POSTAGE & HANDLING_____ *(US: $4.00 for first book & $1.50 for each additional book)* *(Outside US: $5.00 for first book & $2.00 for each additional book)*	☐ Check here if billing address is different from shipping address and attach purchase order and billing address information.
	Signature_____
SUBTOTAL_____	☐ **PAYMENT ENCLOSED:** $_____
IN CANADA: ADD 7% GST_____	☐ **PLEASE CHARGE TO MY CREDIT CARD.**
STATE TAX_____ *(NJ, NY, OH, MN, CA, IL, IN, PA, & SD residents, add appropriate local sales tax)*	☐ Visa ☐ MasterCard ☐ AmEx ☐ Discover ☐ Diner's Club ☐ Eurocard ☐ JCB
	Account #_____
FINAL TOTAL_____ *(If paying in Canadian funds, convert using the current exchange rate, UNESCO coupons welcome)*	Exp. Date_____
	Signature_____

Prices in US dollars and subject to change without notice.

NAME_____
INSTITUTION_____
ADDRESS_____
CITY_____
STATE/ZIP_____
COUNTRY_____ COUNTY (NY residents only)_____
TEL_____ FAX_____
E-MAIL_____

May we use your e-mail address for confirmations and other types of information? ☐ Yes ☐ No
We appreciate receiving your e-mail address and fax number. Haworth would like to e-mail or fax special discount offers to you, as a preferred customer. **We will never share, rent, or exchange your e-mail address or fax number.** We regard such actions as an invasion of your privacy.

Order From Your Local Bookstore or Directly From
The Haworth Press, Inc.
10 Alice Street, Binghamton, New York 13904-1580 • USA
TELEPHONE: 1-800-HAWORTH (1-800-429-6784) / Outside US/Canada: (607) 722-5857
FAX: 1-800-895-0582 / Outside US/Canada: (607) 771-0012
E-mail to: orders@haworthpress.com

For orders outside US and Canada, you may wish to order through your local sales representative, distributor, or bookseller.
For information, see http://haworthpress.com/distributors

(Discounts are available for individual orders in US and Canada only, not booksellers/distributors.)

PLEASE PHOTOCOPY THIS FORM FOR YOUR PERSONAL USE.
http://www.HaworthPress.com   BOF04